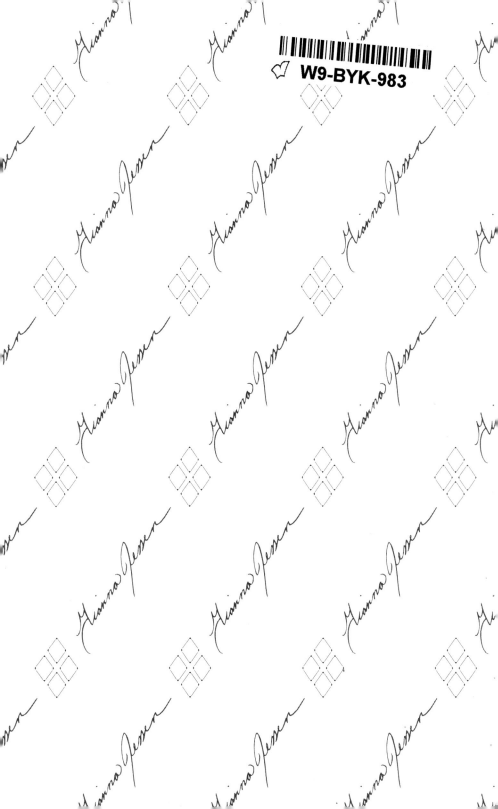

Leanne
BOYD
Please
Return
to
Leanne
BOYD

Gianna's story is more than wonderful—it's prophetic! Having met her as well as heard her, I am delighted to discover the "pure gold" quality of this young woman.

Jack W. Hayford, D. Litt.
Senior Pastor
The Church on the Way

Gianna Jessen is a real spiritual success story. We need the example of her courage as we struggle with the evil of abortion and as a reminder of the glory of the pro-life cause.

Henry Hyde
Member
U.S. House of Representatives

Gianna is a living memorial who allows all to see the millions of children whose lives have been taken by the insanity of abortion. For a brief time, I was in an insane place called Planned Parenthood Federation of America. Gianna's story should be required reading in every high school in America.

LaVonne Wilenken, RN, CNM
Former Planned Parenthood practitioner

Gianna Jessen is living proof that God, the Author of life, will not be mocked, even by those who abort children under the false cloak called choice. Gianna's story must be read by all those who want to understand truth and share in a miracle.

Judie Brown
President
American Life League, Inc.

Gianna Jessen is not only an abortion survivor: she's an abortion conqueror. Gianna has overcome the bitterness of terrible rejection, the limitations of physical handicap, and the contempt of those who would like to silence her. As we climbed up the steep and blustery way to the top of the Cliffs of Moher while witnessing for life in Ireland—me an old man with a cane and Gianna a young girl with a crippled leg—I watched her fall repeatedly on the rain-slicked sidewalk and get up laughing every time: a model for all pro-lifers who face the formidable obstacles ever in our paths. Gianna is a witness to the indomitable human spirit, to the wonder and sanctity of each individual life. Gianna is alive! I thank God for her.

Father Paul Marx, OSB, Ph.D.
Founder and Chairman
Human Life International

Gianna

Gianna

Aborted . . . and Lived to Tell About It

JESSICA SHAVER

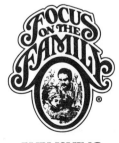

PUBLISHING
Colorado Springs, Colorado

GIANNA

Library of Congress Cataloging-in-Publication Data
Shaver, Jessica.
    Gianna : aborted . . . and lived to tell about it / by Jessica Shaver.
       p. cm.
    ISBN 1-56179-342-6
    1. Abortion—United States. 2. Children, Adopted—United States—Biography.
3. Cerebral palsied children—United States—Biography. 4. Pregnancy, Unwanted—
United States—Case Studies. 5. Abortion—United States—Moral and ethical aspects.
I. Title.
HQ767.5.U5S43   1995
363.4'6'092—dc20
[B]   94-32519
                                              CIP

Published by Focus on the Family Publishing, Colorado Springs, CO 80995. Distributed in the U. S. A. and Canada by Word Books, Dallas, Texas.

Unless otherwise noted, Scripture quotations are from the HOLY BIBLE, NEW INTERNATIONAL VERSION ®. Copyright © 1973, 1978, and 1984 by the International Bible Society. Used by permission of Zondervan Publishing House. All rights reserved.

FRIENDS by Michael W. Smith and Deborah D. Smith. © 1982 Meadowgreen Music Company. Used by permission.

I SEE YOU STANDING © Copyright 1990 by Ariose Music (div. of Star Song) and Mountain Spring Music. All rights reserved. Used by permission of Gaither Copyright Management.

STRENGTH OF MY LIFE by Leslie Phillips © Copyright 1984 by Word Music (a div. of Word, Inc.). All rights reserved. Used by permission.

Editor: Larry K. Weeden
Front cover design: Brad Lind
Cover photography: Reg Francklyn
Photographer for Gianna: Anacleto Rapping

Printed in the United States of America
95 96 97 98 99/10 9 8 7 6 5 4 3 2 1

This is the story of three moms and a baby. It is Gianna's story because she's the girl who survived abortion. But it's also the story of her three mothers:

Tina, her biological mother;
Penny, her foster mother;
Diana, her adoptive mother.

To each of the three, I dedicate this book.

Contents

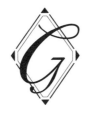

Tragic
Decision
with a
Happy
Ending

chapter 1

April 1977

Tina was trembling when she got off the bus in Los Angeles. Her hands, clutching the small duffel bag in which she had brought her new yellow robe, were clammy. She didn't feel 17. She felt like a little girl again and wanted her mother's hand. But she had been told she didn't need her mother's permission for this, that it was the best thing for her, and that she was being sent here because the other clinic didn't do abortions after the first three months.

It was a sunny, warm April morning, but Tina was shivering, and her hazel eyes were troubled. The bus from Anaheim had taken hours, requiring several transfers. Now she stood before a white, sterile-looking building. AVALON HOSPITAL read the sign at the door. She paused on the threshold, licked her lips, and pushed her wavy, brown hair back from her face. *What am I doing?* she kept asking herself. *I feel so alone.* She wanted someone to tell her secret to, someone to assure her she was doing the right thing.

But someone *had* reassured her. "It's the best thing," she had been told. "We know. We've walked in your shoes."

Tina pushed open the door and entered the building. Beyond the waiting room were two large rooms lined with beds. *Like barracks*, she thought, starting to tremble again. To one side was an examining room. Teenage girls—about 30 of them wearing below-the-knee-length hospital gowns—filled the hall, talking animatedly with each other.

An impatient woman behind a counter held out a clipboard and asked Tina to fill out forms. Name. Date of birth. Date of last period. Tina was genuinely confused about that, but she thought it had been just a little less than three months. (It was actually more like six or seven.) She stole a look at the other teenagers. They were laughing together as if they knew each other well, telling stories about cheerleading camp. *I wish I had someone to talk to.* Tina wondered if the other girls felt as nervous as she did. If so, they weren't letting it show.

There were so many forms to fill out. She knew she should read all the printed material before she signed anything, but she couldn't concentrate. Her mouth was dry, and her mind couldn't make sense out of the words, even though some of them were all capitalized, so she knew they must be important. She noticed something about hospitalization: "IT IS NOT NECESSARY THAT YOU BE ADMITTED TO A HOSPITAL IN THE EVENT OF RETAINED TISSUE. Perforation of the uterus does not require hospitalization. Infection should almost never require hospitalization."

The words swam before her eyes. "We have the greatest experience in the handling of occasional, post-operative problems. . . . It is totally unnecessary for you to seek care at an emergency room or with another physician." *Why are they so paranoid?* the girl wondered. Over and over, the material urged, "Return to us if problems occur."

What problems—and what if they do occur? I have to go through with it. The staff at Planned Parenthood had said so: "You're living with your mother, and she's already on welfare. You can't raise a child." Besides, it wasn't a baby yet. She had felt the growing presence move within her, but they said it was just tissue, just part of her own body.

She signed all the waivers of responsibility and took the clipboard back to the receptionist, who didn't even look up as she said curtly, "Change your clothes in the bathroom, and wait for your name to be called."

Tina started to ask where the hospital gowns were, but the woman's attitude as she bent over her typewriter did not encourage questions. Maybe there were gowns in the bathroom—wherever the bathroom was.

Standing alone against a wall after finding the unattractive, starchy gown and changing her clothes, Tina wished they had let her wear her new robe. It had mandarin orange piping and was silky inside, so much prettier and warmer than the thin, cotton gown. Still chilly, she kept her socks on.

"Tina." The sound of her own name a few minutes later startled her. A nurse was motioning her toward the tiny examining room. Bare walls. Lots of stainless steel. A rather short, physically fit man was at the sink, his back to her, washing his hands. At the nurse's direction, Tina climbed onto the examining table and lay down.

The doctor turned toward her, drying his hands. She searched his face as he felt and measured her rounded stomach with quick, expert movements, but his eyes never met hers.

"Saline," he said when he completed his brief exam. It was the only word he spoke, and as he did, he extended his hand. Tina jerked involuntarily when she saw the length of the needle the nurse handed him.

"Squeeze my arm," urged the nurse, standing now at her side. As the needle went in, a wave of nausea hit Tina, and she squeezed the woman's arm so tightly that her nails pierced the skin.

My body's rejecting this! she thought with panic. *It's not taking it. I'm going to throw up!* She fought to keep still, to stay calm. It seemed to take forever! The doctor's profile—his brown hair neatly trimmed, his face void of emotion—burned into her memory as he leaned over her.

The injection was over. "Drink water and walk," instructed the nurse.

Tina climbed down off the table and walked into the hall. Now *31* women were drinking water and pacing, drinking more water and pacing, waiting for the saline injections to take effect. The day seemed endless as hour after hour passed, and there was nothing to do but wait. Why was it taking so long?

By the end of the day, the hall had almost emptied, and most of the beds in the next room were full. Girls who had come in later than Tina were going into labor, delivering their fetuses, having D and C's (an operation in which the uterine wall is scraped clean) to assure that their uteruses were empty, and being given sedatives and put to bed. The doctor had gone home; so had all but one of the nursing staff.

There was no TV. A girl in the bed nearest the open door had brought a radio. Tina heard her click it on and sample several stations. "You light up my life . . ." sang a clear, comforting voice.

"Turn that off!" snapped the nurse.

The music stopped abruptly.

At last, toward evening, Tina lay down too. She was the only one whose saline injection had not yet taken effect. She must have dozed off, because something woke her in the dead of night.

From the beds around her and in the next room, she could hear only an occasional moan or soft whimper. Most of the other girls were asleep.

Tina had just a low backache, but she felt something warm and wet on her legs. She pushed the buzzer for the nurse, but no one came. She buzzed again, holding the button down determinedly. Finally she slipped out from between the sheets and padded into the hallway. It was empty. Down at the nurse's station, she found someone at last, the nurse on the graveyard shift. The nurse was sitting in a white uniform, arms crossed on her desk and her head on a pillow between them. She was asleep.

The teenager leaned down and touched the nurse's shoulder. "My water broke," she said. "You said to tell you when my water broke."

The woman stirred. "Okay, go back and lie down."

Something different was happening now. Tina felt an urgent need to push, to expel this unknown substance. *Tissue*, the professionals had called it. *Fetal tissue.*

By the time she got back to bed, the muscles in Tina's abdomen were contracting insistently. She had to push—and the nurse still had not come.

Reaching down, she felt the wet, solid curve of a skull. *It's a head!* she thought, shocked. Her heart began to thud in her ears. *How can tissue have a head?* At that instant, a thin, penetrating wail pierced the quiet room. Surrounded by a roomful of women who had delivered limp, lifeless fetuses, a baby girl was making her triumphant, indignant way into the world.

Absorbed in the confusing drama within her mind and body, Tina was vaguely aware of patients around her waking up and screaming for the nurse. With her own hands, she was delivering a bawling, wriggling baby: Eyes scrunched shut, squeezing out real tears. A mouth open, roaring outrage. Tiny shoulders and arms no longer than a pencil, gesticulating. A slippery body, little legs, all perfectly formed. A *little girl—a daughter no bigger than a doll,* she marveled. *This is a baby. What I did was so wrong! How could I ever have let them take this child?*

And then, *This was meant to be.*

Around the two of them, mother and child, pandemonium had broken out. Women were scrambling out of bed and running barefoot to fetch the nurse: "Come quick! She needs you!" Others were sobbing uncontrollably, their eyes wide, their hands over their mouths. But the 17-year-old was in a world alone with her baby. "You're beautiful," she whispered, tracing the small, downy cheeks and stroking the matted, dark hair. "You have the most beautiful face!" The minuscule rib cage heaved with subsiding sobs.

The whole clinic was awake now—even, at last, the nurse on duty. She came at a run, mechanically urging everyone to calm down, trying to regain control. She looked with shock at the little human being cupped in Tina's hands and breathed, "Oh my God!" People were asking her questions, but she didn't seem to hear them.

In the next bed, a girl was sobbing, over and over, "It's a baby! It's a baby! It's a little girl!"

The nurse cut the umbilical cord, lined a bedpan with a blue hospital pad, and laid the baby girl in it. Her middle-aged face looked frightened, and her hands were shaking.

"The doctor," she murmured. "I have to call the doctor! And an ambulance!" She lifted the bedpan carefully and carried the baby away. After a while, she brought papers—many papers—for Tina to sign. "Transfer forms," the nurse said, more controlled now. "Waiver of liability. Birth certificate. Put down that she was born at 4:00 A.M. And give her a name. You have to give her a name."

A *name*, Tina's mind echoed. Exhaustion was bringing with it a sense of unreality. How could she come up, all at once, with a name for a baby she hadn't known she was expecting?

People in white uniforms were arriving—the day shift. It was light outside. A needle slid into the back of Tina's hand, and she felt icy, stinging liquid course up her fingers. Time for her D and C.

She was getting sleepy. A name. She remembered the daughter of a friend of her mother's, a girl named Guyette. She liked the woman, but the name was too masculine. Perhaps just the Guy. And her mother's middle name was Ann. Her thoughts were swirling now. In her mind, Candice Bergen was doing her commercial for Cie perfume. "Cie is me," Bergen was saying.

Guy. Ann. Cie.

Tina filled in the blank before losing consciousness. "Giana Cie." *Cie is me,* she thought as she fell asleep.

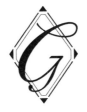

The
Whole
Truth

chapter 2

Christmas 1989

As she rinsed stuffing from her hands, Diana gazed through the window over her kitchen sink. It was going to be another hot, dry Christmas. She didn't have to walk outside to know it was typical Santa Ana weather, with a hot wind blowing in off Death Valley—one of those days her two daughters, especially 12-year-old Gianna (a second *n* had been added to Tina's original spelling, and the G had been softened to sound like a *J*), would want to spend lazing around the swimming pool.

The early morning sun, already warm, slanted through the oaks. It flecked the surface of the pondlike swimming pool with highlights and glistened in iridescent blues and greens on the proud bodies and trailing plumage of peacocks strutting through the woodsy landscape.

As always, Diana took pleasure in the view. She liked living in the country, and Valley Center, California, a community inland and up the hill from Escondido (just north of San Diego), was a wonderful place to live—100 square miles of orange groves and avocado ranches. The house was redwood inside and out, with bay windows framing the trees. Real peacocks strutting in the garden added such an exotic touch! *Eden must have looked like this*, she thought.

Behind her, the turkey sizzled in the big wood stove. *Adam and Eve never cooked their turkeys!* Diana ran the back of her hand across her moist forehead, pulled her brown hair into a ponytail, and fastened it with a rubber band from the pocket of her shorts.

It was probably silly to roast a turkey in a wood stove

11

when she had a perfectly modern oven—silly to radiate all that heat into a house that would be stifling by afternoon anyway—but she didn't care. When her husband, Peter, offered her a vacation in Playa Blanca, she had chosen to buy this 100-year-old, cast-iron Charm stove instead. They had eaten at Ivy House in Laguna Beach that evening, and she remembered taking him by the hand and leading him across the street to Hedges Antiques to show it to him. She still treasured the day they lit the first fire to warm their home. In the winters, when the air was usually crisp and clean, she always cooked on it by choice. Especially at Christmas.

Especially *this* Christmas. Diana sighed and turned away from the window, wiping her hands on a towel. This Christmas, keeping up tradition was vitally important to her. She wanted it to be a wonderful holiday, like those she remembered from childhood. Each year since she'd married Peter, she just held her breath and hoped everything would go all right. So often it didn't. Holidays had become days filled with anxiety, with wondering if she and Peter would get along or if something would set off another argument.

Dené (pronounced Duh-NAY) and Gianna burst into the kitchen, their faces flushed and happy.

"Can I make my cranberry sauce now?" asked Dené. "I promised Natasha I'd go over and see what she got for Christmas." At 16, Dené hadn't yet lost her enthusiasm for getting behind the wheel of her Honda Accord every chance she could.

"Sure, the cranberries and oranges are in the fridge. You know where the blender is."

"What did you put in the dressing this year?" asked Gianna, dragging the wooden stool over beside Diana and climbing onto it.

"Water chestnuts, apples, and raisins." Diana's cheeks were pink and shiny with the heat.

"Mmm." Gianna ran her tongue around her lips and rubbed her stomach. "I can hardly wait."

Diana glanced at the 12-year-old and thanked God silently that with the stress they'd all been under lately, Gianna's eyes could still sparkle.

On the railings outside, Diana had strung colored lights. Inside she had put up wreaths and set out cherished toys from her childhood. There was the 150-year-old china doll in an old-fashioned wicker buggy. There was the teddy bear in a plaid scarf who sat in the little, brown rocking chair Diana's grandmother had brought to California from Missouri by covered wagon when she was four.

If she could keep the house warm and homey, if she could re-create the aromas of Christmas—fresh-cut pine, turkey, sweet potatoes, and pumpkin pie—maybe they would have the storybook Christmas for which she always wished.

There would be just the five of them for dinner this year. Mom lived an hour and a half away with Diana's adopted brothers and four or five foster kids, so she couldn't come. *Why don't I just face it?* thought Diana. *No one wants to come here on holidays anyway, with all the tension between Peter and me.*

Diana shook the thoughts away. "Gianna, you want to set the table?" she asked.

"Sure." Gianna hopped off the chair and limped over to the silverware drawer.

"Dené, when you're through with that—"

"I'm through, but I've gotta go. I promised."

"Okay. Gianna, when *you're* through, could you open the sweet potatoes and the other cranberry sauce? Dené"—as Dené put the blender in the sink and bolted through the doorway—"we'll be eating about 2:00. Be home by 1:30."

Dené nodded and was gone.

When Gianna had pushed the serving dish of sweet potatoes onto the stove and eased the cranberry sauce into a bowl, she said, "Can I go put on my new outfit?"

"If you want to."

Diana was grateful for her daughter's enthusiasm. It was getting harder every year for her to work up any excitement when she had to do all the planning, shopping, and wrapping alone. She hadn't even made cookies this year. She just couldn't bring herself to put forth the effort. But, she reminded herself, straightening her shoulders, she would do what she always did. She would turn a difficult situation into an adventure. She would do it for the girls. They deserved that.

She remembered their animated expressions the night before as they decorated the tree in the open area between the living and dining rooms. Dené's softly rounded face was framed with shiny, brown hair like her mother's; Gianna's freckle-dusted, pixie features were almost hidden by long, blonde waves.

And Grandpa. Grandpa deserved a good Christmas, even if he was never sure why he was getting presents. Diana smiled, thinking of how much fun it was for her and the girls to make everything special for Grandpa. That morning he sat in his recliner in the corner of the big living room, the room that was dark despite all the windows because of the thick stand of oaks surrounding the house. The girls took turns handing him presents and giggling as he asked good-naturedly, "Now who is this for?"

"This is for *you*," they would all answer with a laugh. "It's for you."

Grandpa opened each gift carefully, and there would be gardening tools, a blanket, suspenders, a new cap, or a pocket watch. He always nodded approvingly and said, "This is a most usable item!" The girls would giggle again and go give him hugs. He'd nestle the item back into its box and fold the wrapping paper up with it. That night when he went to sleep, Diana knew he'd have all the presents in bed with him, as he had for all three Christmases he had lived with them—the presents, the paper, and the bows.

As she had every Christmas season throughout this second marriage, Diana shopped for the family by herself. She had stayed up late the night before wrapping presents and filling stockings. Everyone got stockings. Peter and Diana. Dené and Gianna. Grandpa had been especially pleased with the pocket knife in his. And of course the dogs, Lobo and Jake, had to have *their* stockings. This year, a red holiday handkerchief around his neck, Lobo had lunged excitedly at his stocking and snapped up the chili peppers they'd tucked into it to flavor his dog food.

Diana was peeling the potatoes she would mash into creamy mounds when Gianna appeared again in her new clothes.

"Need any more help?" Gianna asked.

"Not right now." Carefully, Diana opened the door of the stove and wiggled a drumstick. "It won't be long." She took a step back, bumping into her daughter, who was trying to peer over her shoulder at the turkey.

"Oops!" Gianna stumbled a little as she backed out of the way. She was quiet a moment, and then she asked, "Mom, why do I have cerebral palsy? I can't help thinking there's a *reason* for it."

Diana stoked the fire in the stove, stalling. It wasn't the first time Gianna had asked about her disability, and Diana had always told her, "You had a traumatic birth. You were premature."

This time, Diana sensed from Gianna's voice that she wouldn't be satisfied with that answer anymore. She glanced over her shoulder and found herself looking into two earnest, blue eyes.

"Mom, I think there's something more you're not telling me," Gianna persisted.

As many times as she had prepared herself for this moment, Diana had not expected it to be here, standing in the kitchen on Christmas Day 1989. Sooner or later, Gianna had to know, but Diana had visualized bringing it up at the beach, on a stroll, or sitting side by side on the white coverlet of Gianna's bed.

It had been easy to talk about adopting her. Diana could discuss the details of the adoption freely and naturally. But this was something else. Once, when Gianna was nine, Diana had been close to introducing the subject, but Gianna was scheduled for a serious surgery, and Diana didn't think her daughter should carry two burdens. How did one explain *this* to a child? Had anyone else ever had to? How would a child—how would *Gianna*—feel knowing this about her birth mother? How would she respond?

I guess she's ready. It isn't my timing, but it must be the Lord's, she thought. As Diana started to break 12 years of silence, she felt a great peace settle on her. *God knows best.*

She turned and looked thoughtfully at her daughter. "Do you really want to know the truth?" she asked.

"Yes!"

"Maybe you'd better sit down."

"No, I'll stand."

"Okay." Diana took a deep breath. "First, Gianna, your biological mother was very young, only 17. She was very scared, without hope or someone to support her. Maybe she had pressure from a boyfriend or her family. She may have felt very alone—"

Gianna beat her to it: "I was aborted, right?"

Diana was taken by surprise. "Yes," she managed.

Gianna was quiet, absorbing this.

"How did you know?" asked Diana.

"I just knew."

"Gianna, I want you to always remember one thing: You were not supposed to live, but God allowed you to have life. You must always focus on the fact that you did not die—you have life. Always rejoice in that gift."

Gianna didn't say anything right away. She was thoughtful, and Diana couldn't read her expression. But when she spoke, it was with her usual perkiness. "Well, at least I have cerebral palsy for an interesting reason." Then, "I'm going to call Jessi and tell her!"

Diana heard her punch her friend's number, pause, and say, "Hey, Jessi, guess what? I was aborted!"

No one mentioned the abortion at dinner, which was mercifully uneventful. Afterward, Peter went out to the barn, and Dené entertained friends by the pool. When Diana had cleaned the kitchen, she went upstairs. Through Gianna's open bedroom door, Diana could see her second daughter lying across the bed, staring into a world of her own.

Diana poked her head in the door. "Are you okay?" she asked.

"I'm fine." Gianna rolled over. "I think it's kind of neat, actually."

"Gianna, I've always told you God has a special plan for your life. You lived. In most late-term abortions, the baby doesn't survive. I've taught you that people who have abortions are deceived. I believe your birth mom was deceived. If she had really known, really understood, what abortion is, she wouldn't have done it." Gianna hadn't moved. "We can talk more about it anytime you want."

That night, when Diana climbed wearily into bed beside her husband, she thought back over the day. Christmas hadn't turned out the way she'd planned. She never would have chosen Christmas Day to tell Gianna about her birth.

But God had chosen the day, she reminded herself, and He knew what He was doing. Maybe she had finally given Gianna the gift she'd wanted most, the gift of truth. God had promised to work all things together for good. As she fell asleep, she prayed that God would bring good even out of this.

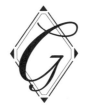

All in the Family

Before that Christmas of 1989, Gianna cried a lot over her biological mother. She thought about her all the time, wanting to know why she gave her up for adoption, wondering what she looked like. But—and this was funny, Gianna thought—once she found out she had survived abortion, she never cried over her biological mother again.

Of course she still had questions: *Why didn't she want me? When she found I was still alive, was she sorry she had the abortion? Does she ever think of me? What's her name? Is she pretty?*

There was no point asking the questions, though, because Diana didn't have the answers. She told Gianna all she knew.

"Your mother was 17," Diana said, tucking her feet next to her on the redwood-frame couch Peter had built. "That's what the medical records say."

Gianna sat at her feet, the sides of her fine hair caught up to the top of her head. Diana handed her what she had received from Orange County Social Services at the time of the adoption. The first item was a birth certificate signed by a doctor who only does abortions. He had not identified the clinic or its location other than filling in *Los Angeles* for both city and county. Peter and Diana were listed as parents.

Then came a page of information about the natural parents: "Natural Mother: 5'5½", 135 lbs., brown hair, hazel eyes. Birthdate 1959. Medical history unknown . . . had had no problems with pregnancy. As natural mother gave date of 1/19/77 as last menstrual period, it was elected to do a saline abortion as natural mother wished to terminate the pregnancy."

Gianna looked up and asked, "What's a saline abortion?"

"That's where the doctor takes some fluid out of the uterus and injects a salt solution into it instead. The baby swallows the solution and goes into convulsions. Usually a few hours or a day later, the mother goes into labor and delivers a dead baby."

Gianna said nothing. Diana wondered if she had been too graphic.

"Gianna?"

"I'm okay, Mom."

"How do you feel about this?"

"Lots of things. I'm not angry at her, really. I don't know how to feel."

Diana also had a sheet from MediCal, a medical assistance program provided through the state of California. A typed note on it, dated July 19, 1977, referred to Gianna as "an infant born ten weeks premature, product of attempted saline abortion." It said she had needed oxygen.

A page of "birth facts" dated 1981 read, "Born during saline abortion, at 29½ weeks gestation. Weight: 1260 grams. Length: 39 cm."

A "Medical Report on Child of Adoptive Family" (1982) said she had been delivered "premature" at six months, weighing two pounds, and that she had been diagnosed as having cerebral palsy. A "Report of Clinic Examination" in 1986 said she was "born at 6½ months gestation following a failed saline abortion."

"The records don't agree on how old you were," said Diana. "One says six months. One says 'ten weeks premature'—that would be about 6½ months."

She went back to the page of birth facts. "This says '29½ weeks gestation.' That's almost 7½ months. I was told you weighed 2.12 pounds and were a little over 15 inches long. Remember those models of babies I use when I give pro-life talks at churches and schools, the ones that show each stage of pregnancy?"

"Is that why you talk about abortion so much, because of me?"

"I started giving talks about abortion a few years before I heard about you—as soon as I realized what women were aborting."

Diana got up and rummaged in a drawer. "Here's a ruler. You were three inches longer than that."

Gianna held the ruler in one hand and added with the other what she guessed would be three more inches. "That's pretty small," she said. She read the next line: "Transferred to Harbor General upon birth, where she remained until discharge 6/6/77."

Diana explained: "When they realized you were still alive, someone must have rushed you to the hospital. We don't know who. You were probably kept in an incubator in the preemie nursery until you were big enough to leave the hospital."

"Is that when I went to live with Grammy?" Gianna asked.

"No, your biological mother kept you for a short time first. Then the Department of Social Services placed you in foster care."

"Why?"

"For not being properly cared for."

Gianna looked at the documents again. "Seven and a half months?" she asked. "But Mom, aren't babies sometimes *born* at seven months?"

"Yes, but it's also legal to abort them at seven months. In 1973, the Supreme Court made abortion legal through all nine months of pregnancy."

"And that's why I have cerebral palsy?"

"We think so. The abortion must have deprived you of

oxygen. The doctors said you would never sit up, much less walk."

"I can do both," said Gianna with pride. "I can play softball and ride a horse, and I even climbed to the top of Multnomah Falls last year."

"That's because Grammy worked with you, massaging your legs and feet and exercising them."

"I remember that."

Before she was "Grammy," she was Penny Smith, a 55-year-old, bespectacled, strawberry blonde in southern California who has always been crazy about babies. She is also Diana's mother.

As an eight-year-old back in Washington, D.C., Penny got her parents' permission to baby-sit an infant who lived across the street. Under the mother's supervision, she played with the baby on the floor of the living room and pushed his stroller up and down in front of the house.

When Penny was 18, a friend's husband died. The friend felt she had no choice but to put all four of her children into a nearby orphanage.

One day, Penny went with her friend to see them. All the kids in the orphanage with no families tore Penny up inside. Local families sponsored some of the children, taking them home on the weekends or bringing them gifts, but a lot of the children had nobody to visit them.

Penny came out of the orphanage that day and got into her friend's car without saying a word, but inside she vowed, *When I get older, I'm going to have a home for children and really give them the best!* She would never be able to speak of the orphanage afterward without struggling against the tears that came to her eyes.

After Penny married and her daughter, Diana, was seven, Penny's husband agreed to adopt a 12-year-old boy and to take in his two younger sisters for "a while." They ended up raising the girls until they were 16.

Penny and her husband took in other children who needed temporary shelter as well. For example, a waitress who used to serve them breakfast at the original Carl's Restaurant after church had some problems with her husband. Penny went to the woman's sister and asked, "Is there any way I can help out?"

"She has five children, and she's trying to find a temporary place for three of them. Maybe you could take one," the sister replied.

Penny talked it over with her husband, and he gave his consent. But when she went to get one, she recalls, "They were all so darling, I said, 'I'll take all three.' " When she brought them home, her husband was flabbergasted.

She laughs about it now. "Man, that was a lot of work! Three boys—a ten-month-old, a two-year-old, and a three-year-old!" That made nine people in the house. But the boys were able to move out when things settled down at their home. "The waitress, who was pregnant, was so grateful for our kindness that she named her newborn after my husband."

Penny got her foster-care license and took in her first official foster baby in 1967, two years after her husband left her for other reasons. Diana was grown and living on her own by then. The baby's name was David, and he was nine months old yet weighed only 8½ pounds. He and his sister had been neglected and were "in a bad way," says Penny. He wasn't expected to live. "All you could see of David were two big, blue eyes."

That afternoon, a friend came over. She was so happy for Penny that she cried, and they spent the afternoon putting little outfits on David that Penny had been saving.

"He loved all the attention and being held," she says. "He was a blessing. Everybody I knew came to see him, and I took him everywhere. The Lord really placed him here." David not only survived, but Penny eventually adopted him, and he became Diana's little brother.

One day in 1978, a caseworker at Orange County Social Services called Penny and said, "We have a little girl who is 17 months old, with cerebral palsy. She has been living in a foster home, but the foster family has six children of their own, and they're expecting a seventh, so they can't keep her any longer. Can you take her?"

As she always did when social workers called to offer her foster children, Penny listened on two levels. On one level, she was taking in what the woman was saying and trying to determine if she could handle one more baby, especially a baby with a disability.

But underneath that listening was an inner listening, or sensing. If this baby was right for her, Penny would know—would feel it—inside. That's how the Lord told her.

She had that inner conviction now. As soon as she could, Penny drove to the foster home to meet the baby, who was chubby and healthy but so limp she couldn't hold herself up. The two took to each other right away, and Penny found herself staying nearly two hours.

She asked questions about cerebral palsy and found out that it's a disorder of the central nervous system resulting from damage to the maturing brain, especially before or during birth. Loss of oxygen during the birth process, a blow to the head—many things can cause cerebral palsy, and the harm can be minor or severe. Gianna's was severe enough that doctors were doubtful she would ever crawl or sit up, much less stand or walk.

The following week, Penny brought Gianna home. They sat in the big rocking chair together, Penny propping the baby upright against her own chest. She read to her and tickled her, and Gianna giggled. There was another faint noise coming from Gianna's throat as well. Congestion of some sort? Penny leaned her head closer to listen. Then she burst out laughing. The baby was humming!

Penny called Diana. "I've got this new little girl, and she's so cute!" she reported. When Diana came to visit, all she could see was curly blonde hair—thin but pretty. Penny had Gianna supported between pillows—a pillow in front of her and a pillow behind—and even so, Gianna was bent double. But for Diana, it was instant love. "Gianna was irresistible!" is how she put it.

The next morning, Penny held Gianna in the big chair and gently rubbed her legs and worked her feet. "You do it, Gianna," she said. "Push against my hand. Push."

Gianna seemed to be trying. Penny let the baby rest for a moment against her chest and gently sang to her. There it was again—the hum.

"That's right!" Penny said. "Sing with me, Gianna! Sing 'All around the mulberry bush, the monkey chased the weasel . . .'" She held Gianna up high. "Kick your feet!"

Gianna hummed and kicked.

"That's a girl!"

Penny sang, and Gianna danced in the air, little by little strengthening the tensed-up muscles in her legs.

Gianna was already in physical therapy at Baden-Powell School three times a week when she came to live with Penny. Penny went to school with her to learn how to do the therapy at home. When doctors told Penny Gianna's limitations, Penny listened politely and then ignored them. She worked daily with the baby, massaging her legs and feet.

At Baden-Powell, the therapist draped Gianna over a large ball and moved it slightly in various directions so she would learn to balance on her stomach. Penny didn't have a big ball at home, but she could hold Gianna up on her toes, push her torso up and down in gentle sit-ups, bend her to each side, and gently stretch the tendons in her legs and ankles. All her medical needs were met by the Crippled Children's Society and MediCal.

When Gianna was 20 months old, Penny recorded in a diary, "We are working with Giana [sic] for better posture, more rotation, balance, and forming better habits of sitting and rising to a standing position."

As Gianna grew, Penny found that she was a worker. Penny helped her with some stretching exercises, and others she was supposed to do alone. She didn't always like them— her muscles were stiff, the exercises *hurt*, and they were lots of work—but she always did them.

One day when Gianna was almost two, Penny found her sitting up all by herself for the first time, legs stretched out and a huge grin on her face. Penny ran for her camera and got a picture, then recorded the fact on the calendar she kept for all her foster children. At the end of each month, she typed up each child's progress, and whenever a child was adopted, Penny presented her new parents with their personal "Life Book," as she called it, and photographs of all their child's milestones.

The baby had a temper, too. She wanted Penny's exclusive attention, and she sometimes got in terrible fights with the other foster child in the house, a four-year-old boy. When she didn't get her way, Gianna would stiffen her body and throw herself backward, bang her head on the floor, and pull her own hair.

Penny had signed a form promising she would never spank her foster children, so she disciplined Gianna by putting her in her room and telling her, "You can come out when you can put on a happy face." Gianna would often cry for a while and then come out of her room on her stomach, pulling herself along with her forearms—and humming, of course. When she got to the kitchen door, she would turn a dazzling face up to Penny. Penny would swoop her up and tell her, "You're a good girl, and what a beautiful smile!"

Gianna loved music. At two, she began singing. By three and a half, she would dance as gracefully as she could in her clumsy leg braces, her face animated, mouth open in wonder.

Diana often came to visit, sometimes with her husband, Peter, sometimes with eight-year-old Dené. All three of them had fallen in love with Gianna.

Once Diana borrowed Gianna for the day. When she got back, Gianna told Penny matter-of-factly, "I have two mommies now—you and Diana." From then on, whenever Diana's family visited, she wanted to go home with them.

The bonding was mutual. Diana told her mother, "I want Gianna to live with me; she's such a sweet little girl."

Penny said, "You should try to adopt her."

"Gianna and Dené really hit it off right away," says Penny. "They were crazy about each other. It really was the Lord working out the whole situation."

When she was three, Gianna stayed with Diana and Peter for two weeks while Penny was out of town. Gianna was already so much a part of the family, it didn't occur to Diana to do anything special with her during that time. Why should they treat her like company? She was just family. They had already bonded at Penny's.

When Penny came for her, Gianna refused to leave. Diana took her upstairs and had a talk with her, and Gianna agreed to go home if Dené could go with them.

They all spent Thanksgiving together. In December, Dené came to visit Grammy for a few days. The girls had a great time. Dené dressed Gianna, did her hair, and helped her practice walking.

In February, Gianna had to have surgery. She spent three days in Children's Hospital, sharing a room with April, a friend from preschool. The operation was done to release the tightness contracting her legs by lengthening— cutting—her Achilles tendon. Penny reported in Gianna's Life Book that "she was cooperative and had a cheerful atti- tude with no fear at any time. . . . The entire experience was a big success."

Afterward, Gianna had to be in casts for ten days. She didn't seem to mind. She walked all over Chuck E. Cheese's in them. When the casts were off, Penny resumed stretching her feet every morning and evening. Now she could stand flat-footed for the first time instead of balancing on her toes.

On April 1, Penny wrote, "Gianna walked without any assistance and without holding on. Feet flat, too! She was so proud of herself." As she grew, her tendon would have to be stretched again and again.

Gianna was four years old five days later. Penny recorded, "Every day she tells me, 'I love Mama Diana. I want her to be my mommy.' Then she'll turn to me and say, 'Let me hug you. I love you.' She is making her own break, and nobody has said a word. It is really the hand of God unfolding her rightful place. We are so happy for her to gain them and for Diana, Peter, and Dené to have such a nice child added to their family. Giana truly loves every one of them."

In May, Penny wrote: "Already she is working out the separation which is taking place. We talk about everything that comes up, preparing her for the move. Her mind is really made up; in fact, she has already made the move in the one important place—her consciousness."

In July: "We are going to miss her. She has been such a joy, and we all love her deeply. Knowing she will be so happy and so well taken care of is a relief. I am so grateful. Seeing her and Dené together is a blessing in itself. The date is set for July 24."

And so, Penny's daughter adopted Gianna, making Gianna's foster mother her grandmother.

"I'll always remember the day I adopted you," Diana told her daughter. "It was wonderful. You were four—this tiny thing with such bright eyes and a big smile—and those big, old, plastic leg braces. You had worked so hard."

They were both quiet a moment, remembering. Gianna had been determined to learn to tie her shoes and dress herself before the adoption—and she wanted to surprise her new mommy by being able to walk without her walker.

On July 24, Gianna pulled her yellow dress on over her head and tied her own shoes. Then she watched out the window until she saw Mommy Diana's car pull up. She started for the door, and almost before Diana was out of the car, the girl with the blue eyes and the blonde pigtails ran stiffly down the driveway and into her new mother's arms—all by herself.

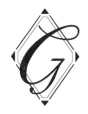

Learning
to Cope

Well, Gianna," said Diana, looking down into the sparkling eyes of the tiny figure strapped into the seat next to her, "where shall we go first? How about the mall?"

Penny had given Diana a large, awkward Pogen buggy big enough to hold the four-year-old, and Diana hefted it out of the trunk when they reached the mall. After setting it up on its creaky legs, she lifted her new daughter into it.

Maneuvering it over curbs was difficult though not impossible. But once they were inside the glass doors, the world began to close in. The elevator was broken, and there was no way that buggy was going to fit on the escalator.

As Diana considered her options—which narrowed down to seeing everything on the ground floor or going straight home—she was vaguely aware of whispers darting like gnats about them.

"Look at that poor little girl in the buggy. She must be at least four years old and can't walk!"

"Pretty little thing, though."

Diana could feel self-consciousness and then anger flushing her cheeks. People walking by—two here, three there, their heads inclined toward each other—would say, "Did you see her?" "Do you think it's polio?"

Is this how it's always going to be? thought Diana. *Never able to do anything without people staring at us?*

At least at home they could overlook Gianna's disability. They didn't actually ignore it, but they took for granted the things she could do, the things she couldn't, and the things she was working hard to learn.

Other adjustments had to be made at home, however. At Grammy's, Gianna had been second in command. Now, besides a mommy, she also had a daddy and a big sister telling her what to do. Eight-year-old Dené was delighted to have a sister sharing her room—until the novelty wore off. Then the periods of togetherness alternated with the squabbles typical between most siblings.

On the third day, Gianna's strong will met its match.

"Honey—" Diana began.

"*Don't* call me *honey!*" Gianna insisted. Hanging on to her walker, the tiny figure glowered up at her mother. "My name's not honey," she said with dignity. "It's Gianna!"

"I will *too* call you honey!" said Diana, just as indignantly. "*Honey* means you care about somebody. You're going to get real used to my calling you honey!" She went on, "I wanted to tell you we're going to have a party to celebrate your coming into our family."

Gianna's wrath immediately turned to delight. "Is Penny coming—I mean Grammy?"

"Sure is."

It was a shower for a pretty big "baby." Penny came and cried. Gianna was in ecstasy. She received all kinds of presents, including a little piano "like Schroeder's." A few years later, a gentleman for whom Diana did some business would give her a real one—a Wurlitzer baby-baby grand—on which she could pick out her own accompaniment when she sang.

Gianna loved to sing. She even sang in the shower, using a bar of soap as a microphone. She had decided, even before she was adopted, to become a professional singer.

Diana's family was able to get away together, all four of them, for a three-week vacation in Colorado. Part of it was a business trip for Diana; she had to close an escrow for her boss, Art Larkin, former CEO of General Foods and Keebler Foods. In exchange, he was letting them spend a week in his mountain cabin at Red Feather Lake. They could fish, hike, and even golf if they liked. The "cabin" was a full-sized house, and it nestled up to a country club that he authorized them to use.

The clear, chiseled peaks, the bristling evergreens, and the crisp autumn weather invigorated all of them. *Southern California doesn't have weather*, thought Diana, closing her eyes and taking in a lung full of cold, smog-free air. She looked at Gianna, perched high on Peter's shoulders, and thought, *If only it could always be like this*. There were bound to be adjustments, she figured, but they would make it.

Late that first afternoon, they visited friends in a nearby cabin. As they chatted, their host built a nest of twigs and crumpled newspaper in the stone fireplace, then lit a fire. No one was prepared for Gianna's reaction. As the wood caught and the flames began to crackle and then roar, Gianna started screaming in terror.

Diana ran to pick her up. "It's okay, Gigi," she said soothingly. "Honey, it's okay! It won't hurt you!"

But the child was hysterical, and Diana had to carry her out into the chilly evening. She walked up and down out of earshot of the cabin, reassuring her, "Honey, that fire won't hurt you. It's pretty, and it will keep us warm."

When they finally went back in, Gianna started crying again, so they had to cut the visit short and go back to their own cabin. Lying awake, Diana shivered just remembering the terror in Gianna's voice.

After their week at the cabin, the family camped for two weeks near Aspen. Each night, Diana would take Gianna in her arms and talk comfortingly to her as Peter built the campfire. She would describe the sounds the fire would make and only take her as close to it as Gianna wanted to go.

Any open fire bothered her. Fires in fireplaces. Campfires. Even fireworks or other loud noises. Diana took her girls to see *Superman*, which opens with a roaring sound, and Gianna shrieked until they hurried her out of the theater.

Finally, Diana took her to counseling and explained her background. Two doctors conferred and concluded, "She is subconsciously reliving the abortion. The roaring and crackling sounds recapitulate the effect of the saline solution as it burned her in the womb."

In most babies aborted that way, the corrosive effect of the salt strips away the outer layer of skin, revealing the raw subcutaneous layer. If the baby swallows the saline solution, it destroys the child's blood-clotting mechanism and produces multiple hemorrhagic or bruise marks. Incredibly, Gianna had no burns or bruises of any kind.

Apart from that one fear, Gianna seemed perfectly happy. The family still lived on three acres near San Diego. Just about the time Gianna moved into her new home, Calvary Chapel leased a small farm at Valley Center and started holding services in its barn. Gianna attended with her family. Later, when the church leaders opened a school in the barn, Gianna entered kindergarten, one of 20 students.

Besides school, there was therapy twice a week and church on Sundays. Sometimes Gianna would get to sing solos in church. She was never happier than when she could sing. She loved to push her walker forward, adjust the mike on the stand (which some adult would have telescoped down as far as it could go for her), and sing praise songs. She had a sweet soprano voice and a natural stage presence; the tiny fellowship at Calvary was enthusiastic. Pastor Craig Landis and his wife, Serena, who taught the school children, were like a second family to Gianna and Dené.

Before Gianna could start first grade there, however, the church school moved to Escondido. Diana signed Gianna up for first grade in Valley Center's public school. On the day school was to start, Diana looked at her second daughter's shining eyes and fine, gold hair in pigtails. She took Gianna's hand and drew her gently to the couch.

"Gianna," she said, "your teacher is going to let each child say what he or she did this summer. When it's your turn, before you say what you did, explain your leg braces. Tell the other kids why you wear them so they won't be afraid of them. Maybe they'll want to touch them or ask you questions about them. Tell them what you have is not catching."

That approach worked—not just in school, but whenever they met strangers. A year later, when Gianna and her mother were waiting for Dené at a gymnastics team practice one day, a small boy came right up to Gianna, put his fists on his hips, and demanded, "Why do you have your shin guards on backward?"

Gianna looked at him calmly and replied, "They're leg braces, and they're not on backward. Would you like to touch them?"

"The school bus is here, Gianna!"

Diana helped her daughter struggle into her backpack and kissed her as she pushed through the door. Dené wasn't there to walk with her to the bus; she had entered Escondido Christian Junior High.

At the foot of the steps, Gianna tripped, landing hard in the middle of a puddle. Watching out the window, Diana gripped the windowsill, making herself resist the urge to run and pick her up. Gianna fell so easily, but Mom wouldn't always be there to soften the fall. Diana knew she had to let her learn to accept falling as a part of life. Gianna was working her way to her feet now, covered with leaves, trying to balance the heavy backpack. Diana's heart was breaking, but as Gianna turned to wave good-bye, she managed a smile and a thumbs-up.

Courage. Life with cerebral palsy required it, and Gianna certainly had it. Diana had never seen a person so determined. In the weeks to come, for example, at recess, Gianna would insist on being included in all the games, even though for her the jump rope had to be held flat on the ground. She wanted to learn, to try. Failure only spurred her on to try anew. She even wanted to be a ballerina.

Oh, thought Diana as the bus rolled out of sight, *I'll bet she forgot to go to the bathroom.* Bladder control was something else affected by cerebral palsy. Gianna had already had more than one accident on the bus.

This time it happened after she got off. "I wet my pants in class," Gianna reported when she got home.

Dené covered her mouth and giggled.

"Didn't you tell Mrs. Martin you needed to go to the bathroom?" asked her mother.

"I tried to, but she was busy."

"What happened?" asked Dené.

"I went all over everything! All over the room!" Gianna started giggling too.

Diana was having a hard time keeping a straight face herself. "We'll *have* to remember to have you go before school" was all she said.

There were lots of bright moments, however. In 1984, Diana and the girls drove to Rancho Bernardo to watch the Olympic torch pass on its way to the Coliseum in Los Angeles. Diana called out to the woman carrying it, "Can one of my girls carry it so we can take pictures?"

"Not me!" said Dené hastily. She was at an age where she didn't want to risk doing anything that might call attention to herself.

The woman graciously stopped and handed Gianna the torch. Diana still has the photograph of seven-year-old Gianna in a teal sweat suit, her hair in braids, proudly holding the torch high as she ran her leg of the journey in braces.

Then there were all the activities after school. Gianna was a majorette and learning to twirl a baton. For Western Days, she walked the entire length of the parade route through town with everyone else, even though the baton teacher brought a wagon for her to sit in when she got tired. She was glad she had gone the distance on her own, but she collapsed from heat stroke at the end of the march and scared her mother to death!

In third grade, Gianna auditioned for a singing group called the Star-Spangled Kids, and she was chosen to sing with them at county fairs, Disneyland, Knott's Berry Farm, and special political events.

Then she joined Christian Youth Theater. She was a munchkin in *The Wizard of Oz*, the studious girl in *Pollyanna*, and she landed the lead in *Alice in Wonderland*. It was a singing and speaking part, and she was a great success, touring with the group to various schools, fairs, and community events.

Gianna had asked Jesus to come into her heart and forgive her sins when she was four. At nine, she rededicated her life to Him. Years later, she would tell radio audiences, "I remember that day when I was nine. I was sitting on my bed in my room and saying, 'Lord, here's my life.' I remember exactly the way the sun was coming in the windows. I believe that God has always been there—I mean, I had to accept Him; I couldn't go into heaven without doing that—but I believe that God just had His hand in the whole situation and put people in my life that directed me to Him."

Waiting for Gianna one day, Diana glanced out the window and saw the school bus coming. She went to the front door and opened it, expecting to see her daughter working her way up the unpaved driveway. But the bus was disappearing in the distance, and there was no sign of Gianna.

Diana ran upstairs for her shoes, grabbed her purse, and dashed out to the car. She drove all the way to school and looked around the lot for a little, blonde girl with a backpack, but she didn't see her. She went inside and asked Gianna's teacher, who was locking the classroom door, if she knew what had become of her.

"Gianna left with everybody else," said the teacher. "I saw her get on the bus."

Now Diana was scared. Had Gianna been kidnapped between the bus stop and her front door? Where would a kidnapper have been hiding on the long, country driveway?

Diana hadn't heard any screams, sounds of struggling, or car engine starting. She drove home with her mind on the calls she would make. Maybe she should notify the police.

As she pulled into the driveway, she saw a forlorn little figure sitting on the front porch.

"Gianna?" she said as she climbed out of the car.

Gianna got to her feet looking weary and disheveled. "Where were you, Mommy?"

"Where were *you*? Weren't you on the bus?"

"I was on the bus, but I forgot where to get off. I was the only one left, and I went past our stop. The driver got mad when I told him. I had to ride all the way to the end, and then he brought me back. It took a long time."

Diana tried to cover her exasperation with a bantering tone. "Good grief, honey, you've been riding the bus all year! You know where to get off! Just pay more attention next time."

She unlocked the door and let the wilted child precede her into the house.

"I'll try not to do it again, Mommy. I *was* paying attention. I just got confused."

The third time Gianna rode past her stop, Diana lost all patience with her. "Gianna, that wasn't an accident! You know better. Why are you doing this?"

"I'm sorry, Mommy."

That night, Diana was helping her with math, trying to teach her how to borrow in subtraction.

"Thirty-six minus eight," she read aloud. "Write that down and we'll do it together."

Gianna made a three and then a nine.

"No, Gigi, not a nine. A *six*."

Gianna erased the nine and tried again. This time the six was backward.

"Stop it, Gianna!" said Diana sharply. "I'm tired, and I don't want you giving me a hard time."

Gianna gazed up at her, her blonde pigtails standing

perkily from each side of her head. "What do you mean?" she asked.

"You know. Now stop it. I'm not in the mood for games."

Gianna looked back at the paper, and Diana sensed that she was genuinely puzzled.

"Do you know what you did, Gianna?" she asked more gently.

"No." Gianna sounded relieved that her mother was beginning to understand.

"You're writing your numbers upside down and backward." Gianna looked at the numbers as if she couldn't see a problem with them. "Here. Look at this six."

Gianna frowned. "Is that backward? I couldn't remember."

"Sure it is. A six goes like this. You've written lots of them."

"I couldn't tell."

A few nights later, they were sitting on the front steps, working on math and getting nowhere. Diana gave up, but in the silence, she remembered a night three years before. "Count backward with me from ten, Gianna," she had instructed. "Start with ten and go down to one."

"Ten . . ." Gianna had started uncertainly.

"What's next?"

"I don't know."

"When you count *up* to ten, what comes right before ten?"

Gianna had thought. "Nine."

"Okay. Ten, nine—then what?"

"Seven?"

"Ten, nine, *eight.* You can do it, Gianna!"

"Ten, nine, eight," she had begun slowly. "Six, three . . ."

I am going to pull all my hair out, Diana had thought. *Just like in the cartoons. My hair is going to stick out all over my head!*

Diana returned to the present. She studied Gianna's math. "No! That isn't right!" she told the little girl. "*Try!*"

Gianna started to cry. "I can't help it! I *am* trying, and I can't *do* it!"

As soon as she could get an appointment, Diana took Gianna to a psychologist. "I'm so stressed out," Diana told the man. "I don't know what to do with her. Everything's going along fine, and then she does these crazy things for no reason. I mean, I know there's a reason. I think she's trying to manipulate me, but I can't figure out why. Sometimes it happens when we're getting along really well."

The man gave Gianna a battery of tests while Diana waited outside the room. When Diana joined the two of them again, he laced his fingers and bored into her eyes with his.

"My dear lady," he said in his Australian accent, "the problem is not the child. The problem is you."

"What do you mean?" she said. "*I'm* not the one riding right on past my bus stop!"

"No, my dear, but your daughter's impairment is not emotional, and it's not deliberate. In reading and vocabulary, she tests at college level! But in mathematics, her sequencing and patterning—her ability to put objects in a given order—is zero."

"It's physical?" Diana asked weakly.

"It's the result of minor brain damage. It's as much a part of the cerebral palsy as her muscle spasticity or her difficulty at times in processing what she's thinking so she can speak smoothly."

"Oh, Gigi," said Diana to her daughter, getting up to wrap her in a hug, "I'm so sorry I blamed you!"

"I *told* you I couldn't help it," said Gianna philosophically.

"You have a wonderful daughter here," said the psychologist. "She thinks very highly of you, and I think you've been doing a good job with her. Just relax and enjoy her."

At the psychologist's suggestion, Diana went in search of

a support group for parents of children with cerebral palsy. Maybe there she could gain a better perspective on what problems and potential Gianna was likely to have. But none of the groups helped, because Gianna's disability was milder than that of most kids whose parents went to support groups, so her problems were different. The parents in the groups Diana visited were looking for respite care or advice on drooling.

That meant she and Gianna would have to learn the hard way just what Gianna was capable of and what she wasn't.

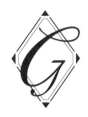

New Surgery and a New Name

Gianna looked tiny and vulnerable on the gurney, her pigtails hidden within a puffy, green medical cap. But she didn't seem to feel the slightest apprehension about her upcoming surgery. After the grueling pre-op tests, surgery almost seemed easy. She joked with nurses and orderlies as she waited to be wheeled down the hall.

She was almost ten. She had undergone two more heel-cord operations since the first one before her fourth birthday, and she had been cheerful and cooperative for each of them—except for the blood tests. She also had plastic surgery to remove mysterious deep scars that had been on the side of her neck ever since Diana had known her.

But this surgery was something new, something called a dorsal rhizotomy. Dr. Warwick Peacock, a neurosurgeon at UCLA Medical Center, had performed it experimentally in South Africa, but Gianna was going to be one of the first children in the United States to undergo it. Her doctor, trained under Dr. Peacock, was Dr. Leslie Cahan of the University of California, Irvine.

"We're going to put you to sleep," Dr. Cahan explained to her, "and test the nerves that control your muscles. The ones that tell your muscles to pull tight when they're not supposed to, we're going to cut. It should give you more muscle control and make it possible for you to walk without leg braces."

To Diana he said, "There is a delicate balance between the messages sent to nerves that control muscle movement. Cerebral palsy upset this balance. Messages that inhibit movement cannot be transmitted, while messages that stimulate those nerves are sent as usual. This means the motor nerves that control muscles are ordered to contract constantly. This is called spasticity. Rhizotomy severs those nerves in the spinal cord that make her muscles contract spastically. Enough normal nerves remain to carry on normal functions."

For six hours, two teams of neurosurgeons alternated to expose Gianna's spine and diagnostically test, with an electric probe, every nerve attached to the spine. All the nerves that tested positive for spasticity were spliced and taken off the spine.

In severe cases of cerebral palsy, doctors have to remove 60 percent of the nerve rootlets that are connected to the spine. In Gianna's case, they only had to remove about 35 percent. But when she was through, she had no muscle control at all. She lay on her hospital bed "limp as a noodle," as Diana put it.

Gianna, thinking back on her hospital stay, remembers it for another reason: "I looked *so ugly!* I was allergic to the tape they put on your face when they put you to sleep with the mask. Oh, I looked—oh!" She shivers.

While Gianna was in the hospital, Diana spent every day with her, even though it meant driving four hours a day. She had to take Dené to a private Christian high school in Rancho California first, drive an hour and a half to Irvine, and then leave the hospital in time to pick up Dené by three o'clock and take her home.

Gianna had brought all her Psalty tapes and videos with her to the hospital. She was there eight days. Every night Diana made popcorn, and Gianna invited all the children in her wing to a party. Children on crutches, children swathed in bandages, children attached to portable IV's—they all came to listen to Psalty. Gianna's stay became a ministry.

She left the hospital flat on her back. The doctors had told her she wouldn't walk for six months, but by the sixth *day*, physical therapists had her on her feet briefly with the aid of a walker. Gradually she sat up, then went to a wheel-chair, then stood up alone a little every day.

Recovery took a full year and a half. Gianna had to learn to sit up and walk all over again. It wasn't practical to have her move back home during this time. For one thing, the Valley Center house wasn't designed for a convalescent. Downstairs was one big room, with no bedroom or bathroom. Also, Gianna needed to make frequent trips back to the hospital for physical therapy, and the hospital was 90 miles away.

Penny's house in Anaheim was much more convenient. It was closer to the hospital and close to Baden-Powell, where Gianna had therapy as a little girl. Gianna could work with her own therapists there—they would even make house calls. So she moved back in with Penny.

As before her first surgery, Gianna had walked on tiptoe before the rhizotomy. As her legs grew, her muscles had resisted until her Achilles tendon was pulling her heel off the ground again. Now, once more, she was able to step flat on her heels. This gave her better coordination. She moved more easily and didn't fall down quite so much as before. Diana home schooled Gianna while she was getting stronger, and she was back on her feet in time to sing in the talent show right before her sixth-grade graduation.

The family celebrated Gianna's graduation at Penny's. That night also meant her return home to Valley Center after the year-and-a-half stay with Grammy.

The separation wasn't painless, but Gianna had a new sense of knowing where she really belonged, and she was eager to return home to her parents, friends, and country house. No one foresaw the storm clouds gathering over her family or knew that this would be her last summer to romp in the hills around her home.

Summer was a time of expectation. Gianna would enter junior high in the fall, and Dené was going to be a senior in high school. The girls grew closer and spent most of their time catching up on last days together at their beach house on the Oceanside strand. They also talked about the cold distance developing between their parents.

September arrived hot and dry, school started, and Gianna made new friends. The following spring, Peter asked for a separation.

Reeling, Diana asked God to show her where to move. She drove up and down the Orange County coast, not feeling led to return to Laguna Beach, where she had lived for almost 13 years.

As she cruised along the coastline, she listened to praise music over her car radio. After one particularly soothing song, the announcer said, "You're listening to KWVE—K-WAVE, San Clemente—the wave of living water."

A small voice in Diana's heart repeated, "San Clemente." She knew where she would find a new place for her family.

Gianna helped in the house hunting, and the Lord provided a place large enough for all of them: Diana, Dené, Gianna, Grandpa, and Judy Devish, who helped care for Grandpa each day and who agreed to come and assist until the family settled in. There was also a yard for their dogs.

Diana clung to God as she entered the most difficult two years of her life. Separation was not what she wanted, but Peter was adamant. Friends offered financial support and provided meals and lots of love. Diana's mom and older brother helped with rent and food, too.

Diana worked wherever she could. She helped with SHARE, a community food program in San Diego, but the commute was too long. She served on the staff of a conservative politician for a while. She worked in case management with senior services at a local senior citizens' center. Thinking back, Diana says, "I don't know how we lived. We lived frugally." Her first husband, Dené's father, paid for Dené's college expenses.

Grandpa finally settled down and became acclimated to

his new environment. Judy returned home, and Diana decided not to replace her with additional help. They needed time to adjust, heal, and pray. Gianna and Dené entered counseling. The family found a new church, Calvary Chapel Pacific Hills, near Laguna Niguel.

Maybe, Diana thought, *this is the time to talk to Gianna about changing names.* She had two reasons for thinking this was important. First, throughout Gianna's childhood, Diana had told her, "Someday you'll be a great singer, and you'll have a stage name." As they drove to church or school, the two of them would think up names. "Gianna Giovanni," suggested Diana once, and they both giggled.

Second, when Diana got involved in the pro-life movement and became a lightning rod for hostility from pro-abortionists, she realized there was a more serious reason for Gianna to have a stage name. Pro-choice advocates had criticized Diana for bringing to her group presentations jars containing fetuses at various stages of growth, preserved in formaldehyde, to give visual proof that what was aborted was a real baby. What would they do once they—and Gianna herself—found out that Gianna had been aborted and lived to tell about it? Gianna would be an even greater target, concluded Diana. A pseudonym would help protect Gianna from threats or actual attacks.

She broached the idea to her daughter. "This might be a good time for you to pick the name you'll have as a singer," she said.

"Okay," Gianna replied. "I want a name with Jessi in it. Something like—Jessen."

Diana wanted a clean break with Peter, so she said, "I'm going to change mine, too. I'm going to be Diana DePaul." Officially, they would both hold Peter's name for passports and legal documents. But they would keep that surname private. Dené, who had never shared her stepfather's surname, would keep her biological father's name.

Later, Diana regretted choosing different surnames. It

caused confusion. Sometimes people who heard Gianna speak or sing assumed she had kept her birth mother's surname. More than that, to the public, Diana felt, the different names seemed to separate the two of them when they weren't separate at all.

Late in March 1990, Gianna entered Shorecliffs Junior High in San Clemente. She missed her best friend, Jessi, and hoped to find some new friends there. It had been hard for Diana to move, but she felt getting away from Valley Center was the best for the girls, and they had pleaded with her to leave. Moving had been a good decision, she concluded.

Dené, who had left home first, was living with family near Lake Elsinore and wasn't ready to leave them. Gianna missed her, too, and would wander into the new bedroom that was to be Dené's and ask God to bring her home.

That prayer wasn't answered until a week before Dené's senior prom. Dené had rededicated her life to Christ and had been accepted to Calvary Chapel Bible College in Twin Peaks, where she began classes in late June.

Jessi spent most of the summer with Gianna, and her presence filled the void Dené left. The girls split their time between the beach, Gianna's room, and Disneyland. They dreaded the end of summer.

Diana spent hours in court and at her attorney's office, fighting a battle she didn't want to fight. Gianna heard from her dad once and then not at all. She felt rejected. But gradually, Diana and her daughters began to recover and lose some of the numbness from the family's deterioration.

Summer slipped into fall, and Gianna entered eighth grade at Shorecliffs in September.

"Well," asked Diana not long after the school year started, "how do you like eighth grade?"

"I don't," said Gianna, dropping her book bag onto the kitchen counter.

"What happened?"

"Oh, the kids I talk to in class act like they don't know me at lunch."

"How about your teachers?" asked her mother.

"They're okay, but, well, it's hard having classes in different rooms. I was late to everything, and the teachers all tried to be, like, real understanding of me. They said I could leave class five minutes early so I'd be on time to the next one."

"That was nice of them."

"But *lots* of kids were late. They got lost and stuff, you know. Why did the teachers have to single me out? And they said, 'We'll give you a book buddy,' you know, someone to carry my books between classes. I've carried my own books since kindergarten!"

"It'll get better," Diana assured her. "Give it some time."

But the situation didn't improve. Gianna came home in tears more than once. "My friends hang out with me outside of school," she said, "but they don't want to be around me in school. They leave me at the lunch table all alone."

"Maybe we should just go back to home schooling, like after your surgeries," suggested her mother. "Why don't we go talk to the principal about it?"

Diana set up an appointment, and at the scheduled time, the principal and school psychologist welcomed them into the office and offered them a seat. "What can I do for you?" the principal asked.

Gianna burst out, "I want to be home schooled."

Diana described some of what Gianna had been through.

The principal was sympathetic. The psychologist was apprehensive. He turned to Gianna and said, "I think we can help. We can get some people to hang out with you—some volunteer friends."

"I think not," said Diana. She thanked them as civilly as she could and ended the interview.

Gianna left the office steaming. By the time they got home, she was boiling over. "Dené!" she exclaimed the minute she heard her sister come in the front door for a weekend home from college. "You won't believe what my principal said today! We went to ask if I could be home schooled because kids won't hang out with me, and he said, 'We can get you some volunteer friends.' Can you believe it!"

"That's low," agreed Dené. "So are you going to let her stay home, Mom?"

"You'd better!" said Gianna. "I'm not going back there!"

"I think it might be better for her," admitted Diana.

That evening, Gianna's anger gave way to tears. She sobbed into her mother's lap for a long time. At last she raised her flushed, wet face to ask in a small voice, "When's God going to heal me, Mom?"

Diana stroked her hair. "Gianna," she said, "it might not be God's will to ever heal you, but He is going to use you in a *very special* way."

"*What* way?"

"I don't know. All I know is that He saved your life for a reason." Diana looked at her daughter tenderly. "He wants to do something extraordinary through you, and He'll show you what it is when He's ready."

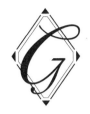

Her First Public Testimony

Soon after Gianna learned she had been aborted, Diana's good friend Bev Cielnecky, national president of Crusade for Life, called to ask if Gianna would be the keynote speaker at their Mother's Day banquet. It would be a small gathering, she explained, for staff and supporters. Bev and her husband, Bob, had been active in pro-life causes for 15 years.

"Do you think she'd be willing to talk about being aborted?" Bev asked. "I mean, since she knows about it now? She would be such an encouragement to our people, a living witness that abortion is about real people and that their efforts to stop it are important."

"I don't know," said Diana. "I'll ask her."

Gianna's answer was immediate: "Sure—if I can sing."

On the night of the banquet, after everyone had been seated and the food had been served, Bev Cielnecky announced, "Four years ago, Penny Smith was our mother of the year—some of you remember. She told us all about her foster children, and especially about one named Gianna. Penny's daughter Diana adopted Gianna, and Diana was at that meeting, too, passing around pictures of this tiny girl with hair like golden cotton candy."

There were murmurs of "Oh, yes!" and "Is this her?"

"Well, this is Gianna. Her mom tells me she's been singing in public since she was three years old!"

Gianna limped to the front of the room, a grin on her face. She wore a loose yellow shirt, caught up at the waist with a cross, and a red print skirt.

Prying the microphone loose from its stand, she greeted the group easily: "Hi, my name is Gianna Jessen. I guess some of you know my mom, Diana." She gestured with her free hand. "She's been working for pro-life for a long time."

Gianna moved freely back and forth across the front of the room, her eyes sparkling. She obviously enjoyed being there, but Bev noticed that Diana watched apprehensively. Gianna was paying scant attention to where she placed her feet, and there were microphone and speaker cords that could easily trip her up and send her sprawling.

"I'm glad to be here," Gianna continued, "and if my mom will start the tape . . ." Professional contemporary background music began pouring through the loudspeakers. "This song is one of my favorites. It's by Amy Grant."

When Gianna started singing, Bev forgot about the concern in Diana's eyes. Gianna's voice was a young, higher version of Amy Grant's, and she had adopted the singer's nuances and pacing. But there was a stage presence about her, a personality, all her own.

She ended a little breathless and shook back her hair. "I just love Amy Grant," she said. "I want to be just like her, and I hope sometime I can meet her." She sang again and waited till the applause died down to tell the group, "I want you all to feel comfortable, so if you have any questions or anything, go ahead and ask."

"I have one," said a woman. "You have a beautiful voice. Do you take lessons?"

"Not yet, but I'd like to."

Bev asked, "Why do you use the name Gianna Jessen?"

"Oh, that's my stage name," said Gianna. "I picked that name for Jessi Oliver, my all-time best friend!"

Then, for the first time, she spoke publicly about being aborted.

With the microphone cradled in her hands, Gianna explained informally, "I'm adopted. My biological mother was 17. When she was seven months pregnant, she chose to have a saline abortion. But by the grace of God, I survived." She smiled.

"I forgive her totally for what she did. She was young, and she probably had no hope. She didn't know what she was doing.

"As a result of it, I have cerebral palsy—but that's okay, because I have God to keep me going every day. I'm not saying that it's easy going through every day, but He's always there. He'll always be there for me as well as for you.

"This last song I want to sing is called 'Friends.' It's by Michael W. Smith, and I want to dedicate it to all the little babies who die from abortion every day—because they *are* my friends, and I'm going to see them in heaven some day."

She began to sing, and the room was filled with her clear, sweet voice:

> And friends are friends forever
> if the Lord's the Lord of them,
> and a friend will not say "never"
> 'cause the welcome will not end.
> Though it's hard to let you go,
> in the Father's hands we know
> that a lifetime's not too long
> to live as friends.

FRIENDS by Michael W. Smith and Deborah D. Smith
Used by permission.

As Gianna finished and lowered her eyes and the microphone, the room was silent while women wiped away tears. Then the audience burst into sustained applause. Afterward, people surged forward to hug her and shake her hand, telling her "I'm glad you survived!" and "I'm so happy you're alive!"

As the crowd thinned out, Gianna turned to go. A woman who had been standing at the fringes of the crowd stepped up to her tentatively.

"I had an abortion," she admitted in a low voice, searching Gianna's face. "Nobody knows. I've confessed it to God, but I still feel guilty."

"You didn't know what you were doing," said Gianna sympathetically.

The woman reached out and stroked Gianna's cheek. "I had to touch you," she said, sighing deeply. "I have longed to hold my baby and tell her that I was sorry. Somehow, touching you, having you say you forgive your mother, makes me feel"—she choked back a sob—"maybe *she* would forgive *me!*"

"She would," said Gianna earnestly. "I *know* she would."

The woman's tears were running freely now. "I've had this bottled up for so many years." She wrapped her arms tightly around Gianna and pulled her close. "Thank you! Thank you!"

Gianna returned the hug.

Then, as the woman held Gianna at arm's length and gazed at her again, Gianna said with conviction, "You will see her in heaven."

The woman took a deep, ragged breath, letting go of years of pain. "Thank you. You have helped me *so much!* God bless your ministry." She gave Gianna's hand one quick squeeze and walked away.

And that was the beginning.

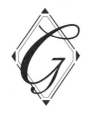

Into the Spotlight

chapter 7

Driving into the hills of San Clemente, the reporter steered her car into a cul-de-sac and parked. Across the valley ahead of her was a green-gray ridge patched with red-tile rooftops leading like stairsteps down to the misty Pacific. The sky was clear; at least in this part of Southern California, stars would be visible at night.

Gianna's family lived in a fawn-colored, two-story, clapboard house—a comfortable home, perhaps 3,000 square feet, with gables like circumflexes over some of the windows. The yard was nicely manicured but dry, a reminder that this was high desert, along a coastline where palm trees and cactus seem paradoxical neighbors.

At her knock, the reporter could hear barking and scuffling, and a girl's voice called breathlessly, "Sorry! Just a minute!" The door opened awkwardly; Gianna—this must be Gianna—was bent over and using her free hand to hold back three eager dogs. She had to struggle to keep them from knocking her off balance.

At last Gianna stood up and grinned. She was 13 years old, with wavy, shoulder-length, blonde hair, blue eyes, straight teeth, and a clear complexion. Rings adorned almost every finger, and she had four earrings in her ears. She wore jeans and a Washington Huskies T-shirt. Behind her, Diana, the woman who adopted her ten years before, invited the stranger in.

The reporter found herself seated on a couch in a split-level living room built around a brick fireplace and furnished with antiques, pine cones, and peacock feathers in a vase. A glass of lemonade was in her hand, a golden cocker spaniel pressed against her left hip, and a full-grown black Lab draped contentedly across her lap.

"All three dogs were abandoned," Diana was telling her. "Come here, Sally! Lobo, get off her!"

Neither dog even rippled a muscle.

"I have the spatula," Diana threatened them both, brandishing it. But she was smiling in spite of herself, and they paid no attention.

Gianna sat on the beige carpet, and as she talked about the Christmas Day when she learned she was aborted, the reporter was struck first by her animation—she was a kid in the freshest, most unsophisticated and fun-loving sense of the word—then by her candor, and finally by her lively sense of humor.

"How do people respond at your concerts when you say you were aborted?" The reporter had turned on her tape recorder, and her pen was poised over a clipboard.

"They cry," said Gianna simply. "People come up and tell me they're glad I survived. Some women who have had abortions say they're sorry they did. I always tell them I understand, because they didn't know what they were doing. I'm not trying to put a guilt trip on them."

She struggled to her feet. "I'll show you a letter I got. It's from Tricia, a year older than me."

She unfolded the letter as she brought it and read it aloud when she had settled back onto the carpet. "In one week, 14 friends changed their mind about abortion since I showed them your picture. One girl I know is a freshman [in high school] and has already had three abortions and is now one month along, pregnant again. She was going to get an abortion, but one of my friends told her about you. Now she is keeping her baby."

She talked about Penny, her foster mother, and about her surgeries.

"You're—how old?"

"I'm going on 14. My birthday's in April." Gianna thought for a moment and turned to her mother. "If I was aborted," she asked, "how can I have a birthday? How can it be my *birth*day when I wasn't born?"

Diana smiled and shrugged. She had been rummaging through a drawer for something. Now she held out several sheets of paper to the reporter. "Here are the hospital records they gave us when we adopted Gianna. They don't agree about how far along the pregnancy was. You can have this one about the birth mother. According to her, she was only three months along, but they told us Gianna was 2.12 pounds, and that's a third-trimester baby. I tore off the case-worker's name at the bottom, because that should probably be kept confidential."

"The abortion caused her cerebral palsy?"

"Yes. It caused a lack of oxygen."

Gianna put in, "I don't feel I have a disability except when I get out of bed in the morning and fall right over. It's funny—you should see it. No broken bones yet, but I've taken some tumbles. Once I was a munchkin in *The Wizard of Oz*. All the cast were sitting on the stage. I came down from the stage, and a little boy thought I was a real munchkin and jumped on me. I tumbled right over and hit my head on the cement floor. My mom said she could hear it all the way across the room. No concussion or anything, so it was a neat experience!

"When my brain sends messages to my legs, it's not the same as when yours does. It just gets kind of complicated. But I'm normal. I'm just a normal teenager. I like talking to my friend Jessi on the phone. I like New Kids on the Block and movies and crafts. I like reading, softball, baking, hanging out at the beach, walking on the pier—"

"She's a whiz at Nintendo," volunteered her mother.

"But I especially like music. Music is me. I love it. I like writing songs, I like to sing, and someday I'd like to record songs I've written."

"Who else is in your family?"

"I have a big sister, Dené, except she's not home much now because she goes to Calvary Chapel Bible College in Twin Peaks. She's 18. There's my mom—"

Diana added, "My husband—my *ex*-husband, Peter—used to live with us. We had a lot of problems. The day I thought he was going to suggest we go for counseling, he said, 'I want a divorce.' "

Gianna, who had been watching her mother, turned back to the visitor for clarification. "Do you mean, who's *actually* part of our family or who *lives* here?"

"Is there a difference?"

Diana laughed. "I get strays," she explained.

"Robyn lives here," went on Gianna. "She's an unwed mother with a one-year-old, and she's pregnant."

"And the dogs," the reporter prompted.

"And the dogs. And Grandpa, of course."

"Grandpa?"

An old, wizened man shuffled out of a bedroom. Diana jumped up. "What do you need, Grandpa?" she asked.

"DosveeDEENya," said Grandpa. "DosveeDEENya."

"He does that all the time," said Gianna, giggling.

The frail, bowed figure was wearing a gray-and-orange-striped shirt, black sweat pants, a beige cap, and white tennis shoes. When Diana came back, the reporter asked her, "Isn't that Russian for *good-bye*? I thought it was supposed to be pronounced dosveeDONya."

"I guess it's Russian," Diana said. "That's where he's from, Russia. He speaks seven languages fluently. He came to the United States in 1913, through Ellis Island. To this day, he still complains they never gave him a receipt for his $25 to get into the country!

"He's not really our grandpa. His name is John Ostro. We found him in an alley five years ago, when he was 96 years old."

"In an alley?"

"Yes. It was 105 degrees, and I was running an errand for a

political candidate. I had seen Grandpa before, standing over a Dumpster, going through the trash looking for food. This time, I asked him if he wanted to come home with me, and he said yes. I had to keep the car windows rolled down all the way home because of the smell—and the flies were terrible!

"The first time I cleaned him up, I couldn't believe what I was doing! He had messed himself, and he was filthy. And he had bronchitis. He had lived on the street for ten years. I taught him to live in a house, but he still lines his bed with newspapers for warmth. It's a street habit."

The phone rang in the kitchen. While Diana was answering it, Grandpa shuffled into the living room. "I'm an explorer," he informed the reporter.

"That's wonderful."

He worked his way slowly out of sight.

When Diana came back, the reporter said, "So he's 101? He must have some incredible stories."

"He would if he could remember them. At first he told me he was a missionary. He loves the Lord."

Grandpa "fell through the cracks" of social services, she explained. Diana knew all about those services. She was a case manager for the elderly at the senior center in Laguna. She had been able to track down John's sister, then in her nineties, and arrange for her to come see him. He also had a brother in Argentina who was 104 the last they knew.

"My grandfather gave me a love for older people," said Diana. "And my great-grandmother lived near us with my grandparents till she died at 98. I remember her stories about growing up in Missouri, hiding under the porch from the Indians."

"And the dogs? Tell me about the dogs."

"They were all strays. I found Lobo the year before I found Grandpa—in a grocery store. He was six months old, and he belonged to some migrant workers, but he got left behind when they got arrested.

"I brought him home, and he chewed every stick of furniture in the house—chair rungs, table legs, French doors. Peter built our redwood couch—"

"And Lobo ate it," said Gianna with a laugh.

"But he wouldn't eat dog food. All he knew was tortillas, refried beans, and salad."

"He loves tomatoes and cucumbers," added Gianna.

"He's the only dog I know with onion breath!"

"Dené finally got him to eat dog food by covering it with salsa."

The phone rang. Diana jumped up again.

"Zing one," Grandpa mumbled. "Zing two."

"That's right, Grandpa," Gianna called to him cheerfully, adding for the sake of the guest, "He likes to count the rings. I hope it's someone who wants me to sing!"

"Is that what you want to do most, sing?"

"Yes!" She squeezed her shoulders together, savoring the thought. "I wish I could give a concert every night!"

The interview with Gianna, "A Survivor of Abortion Grows Up," appeared on the opinion page of the *Orange County Register* a week later, on January 22, 1991. The article read in part:

"Gianna Jessen is going on 14, but the date in April that she will celebrate as her birthday isn't really her birthday, because she was never born. She was aborted. . . .

"Whether Gianna's birth mother was pregnant 24 weeks or 26 or 29½ (the medical records conflict), the abortion was legal under Roe v. Wade, the Supreme Court ruling handed down 18 years ago this month. Her doctor injected a saline solution into her uterus and expected her to deliver a dead fetus the next day. Instead, she delivered a live baby. Gianna weighed two pounds . . ."

It closed with the quotation from Gianna's fan letter.

Almost immediately, Gianna started getting calls. Someone from the National Right to Life office wanted her to speak and sing at their annual convention coming up in July. "The 700 Club" wanted her on their program in

September. A Catholic group invited her to speak in Washington, D.C., during the National Week of Prayer in October.

Soon Gianna was receiving so many invitations that Diana had to retain a Christian agent to screen and keep track of them. Gianna was starting to see her dream fulfilled. By September, she would be singing somewhere almost every night.

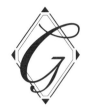

The
Politics
of Abortion

On May 8, 1991, Gianna flew with her mother to Montgomery, Alabama, to speak before the Health Committee of the state legislature. The committee was considering a bill allowing abortions only for women who were victims of rape or incest or whose lives were endangered by the pregnancy. Those cases total perhaps 2 percent of the 1.6 million abortions done yearly in the United States.

The bill made exceptions for the delivery of babies prematurely to preserve the health of the mother or the child. Doctors could be held criminally liable for abortions; pregnant women could not.

Before the vote, arguments on both sides of the bill raged in the local newspapers. Carrie Gordon, executive director of the Alabama Pro-Life Coalition, estimated publicly that if passed, the bill would stop all but about 600 of the 30,000 abortions performed in Alabama each year.

Diane Derzis, director of the Summit Medical Center abortion clinic in Birmingham, disagreed. "There would not be a single abortion in this state," she said. There would be no *legal* abortion, other pro-choice proponents declared, but women would seek illegal abortions or commit suicide.

David Smolin, law professor at Cumberland Law School in Birmingham, supported the bill as a trial case that might ultimately lead the Supreme Court to reverse its decision in Roe v. Wade. Opponents argued that its language was so stringent that it could be interpreted to prohibit Caesarian-section deliveries, low-dose birth-control pills, or intrauterine devices.

But all agreed that sympathies within the House lay with the bill. "Outside of a miracle, it will pass the House," Derzis complained to the *Mobile Press*. "It's touch-and-go in the Senate."

Into this cauldron of heated public opinion, Gianna stepped, offering the simplicity of herself. It was the first time she had given her talk to a group that included people on the other side of the issue. She was scared, but she wanted to tell her story, to put a living, human face on abortion.

More than 100 people had gathered in the committee hearing room, and many more were listening to the debate from the Senate chambers over the public address system. Gianna appeared before the committee in a black dress with white polka dots.

When invited to speak, she walked to the microphone and described simply how her birth mother had chosen abortion and how she had been delivered alive. "The abortionist told my mom, 'There is not a life here.' But there is," she said. "I am not a blob! I don't like to be called a blob. I wouldn't call you a blob!

"I just want you to think about how many other babies go to heaven before they even get a chance to live. I like to run. I like to jump." She spread her arms. "I am a person! That's all I have to say."

Shaking inside from a combination of excitement and fear, Gianna made her way back to her seat near the front of the room. She was about to feel the wrath of pro-abortionists for the first time in her young life.

The very next witness demanded, "What about handicapped children?" Her question was directed at the committee, but she turned to face Gianna as she said it. Her eyes bored a challenge into Gianna's as she proclaimed, "Children with disabilities are a burden to society!"

The woman's remarks shocked Gianna, and she shivered involuntarily. *Would people like this actually prefer that I had never been born?* The idea stunned her. *Do they really think that having survived abortion or having a handicap makes me worth less than others?* The depth of animosity toward her that she felt in that moment made her both more determined about the pro-life cause and more wary of its adversaries.

Another witness, Montgomery gynecologist Judi Jehle, built on Gianna's remarks: "I wish I had a nickel for every time I make a visit to the emergency room to help someone with postabortion complications. Many times patients have told me, 'I didn't know the tissue removed was alive—I didn't know there was a heartbeat.' " She added that based on her observations as a doctor, she believed regard for the sanctity of life had diminished in the United States since Roe v. Wade.

The Rev. Doak Mansfield of the Unitarian Universalist Church of Huntsville dismissed arguments against abortion as religious. "For one religious interpretation to become law is un-American," he said. "Let those who oppose reproductive freedom teach, preach, and educate from their religious understanding."

That night, the *Alabama Journal* quoted from Gianna's short speech. Two Alabama newscasts that reported on the hearing included clips of her. On News Center 5 in Mobile, a female newscaster announced, "Supporters of a strict abortion bill say that it will pass the full Alabama House just as quickly as it did a legislative committee.

"One person who hopes the bill becomes law is 14-year-old Jenna [sic] Jessen. Jessen says she was aborted by saline solution in the third trimester of her teenaged mother's pregnancy. She was born alive, she weighed two pounds, and she survived."

The scene cut to Gianna, now wearing a blue, flowered dress with a square neck, seated with plants behind her. "As a result of the abortion, I have cerebral palsy," Gianna said.

"The doctors said I wouldn't do anything—I wouldn't sit up, I wouldn't crawl, I wouldn't walk. But I can—" Curiously, though her lips continued to move, the rest of the sentence was muted. It wasn't hard to read the words the station censored: "and I praise God for that."

The newscaster continued, "Jenna has testified before state legislative committees"—actually, this was the first one—"asking for an end to abortion on demand."

That same night, the newscaster on a Birmingham television station announced, "A bill to ban abortions in Alabama made its way out of the House committee today after emotional testimony. A 14-year-old girl who survived her mother's abortion testified in favor of the measure. Gianna Jessen was aborted by saline solution in the third trimester of her teenage mother's pregnancy. To a doctor's surprise, Gianna was born gasping on that saline solution."

Gianna was then shown standing at the microphone before the committee in a brief clip from her testimony.

Newscaster: "After Jessen's comments, pro-choice advocates voiced strong opposition to the measure." Planned Parenthood Director Larry Roddick then was on the screen saying, "This bill is mean and hurtful. It gives the government the power to dictate reproductive options. It will endanger the life and the health of Alabama's women and the welfare of their families."

Newscaster: "The abortion bill now goes to the House."

The following day's *Montgomery Advertiser* reported that the state legislative committee had "overwhelmingly approved" the bill. "The 11-2 vote by the House Health Committee came after emotional testimony from a 14-year-old girl who survived her mother's saline abortion."

Looking back on the bill he sponsored, Alabama Representative Jim Carns says, "Gianna had a very big impact on the committee. I was at both committee hearings, and the most potent thing I heard all the way through the proceedings was her testimony. You can't argue against a real, living human being."

The bills opponents, however, could and did kill the bill that would have protected the lives of others like her. It passed the full House 69-30. It passed the Senate Health Commitee. But pro-abortionists kept it from reaching the floor of the Senate for debate, and it died at the end of the legislative year.

Later in that same month of May 1991, Gianna got her first opportunity to sing and speak overseas. Jorge Molinero, a reporter for Spain's *Palabra* magazine, had seen her at an event in Santa Clara, California, earlier in the year and extended the invitation to his country.

In anticipation of the trip, another reporter interviewed her for *¡HOLA!*, Spain's counterpart to *People* magazine ("only bigger," according to Diana). That issue of the magazine, which included a five-page spread of color photos plus questions and answers, was on the newsstands when Gianna and Diana stepped off the plane in Madrid.

While in Spain, Gianna performed in Madrid, Barcelona, and Seville. Everywhere she went, she won the hearts of the people, who were warm and gracious in return. She received extensive media coverage, giving her the chance repeatedly to tell her story of surviving abortion and forgiving her birth mother. At a girls' school in La Florita, Gianna expressed the core of her message when she said, "If you don't have forgiveness in your heart, you won't be very happy, because your heart will get hard."

The tour was a great success in every respect except for one: The whirlwind schedule, culture shock, and jet lag combined to give Gianna a turbulent stomach throughout the trip. Memories of the people and their kindness, however, were more than enough to make up for the temporary discomfort.

Such kindness would be sorely lacking a month later,

when Gianna spoke out for life in her own home area of Southern California.

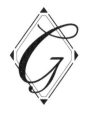

Shouted
Down
in L.A.

chapter 9

N one of Gianna's previous appearances, even the one before the Alabama legislature, prepared her for the heckling she had to endure before the Los Angeles County Board of Supervisors.

One of the most powerful groups in the country, the five supervisors manage a $13 billion budget—larger than that of 37 *states*. They serve ten million constituents, or more than the populations of 46 states.

On July 9, 1991, they were hearing testimony, first against and then for, testing the controversial abortion-causing pill RU-486 on Los Angeles women. In France, 100,000 women had used it to induce early abortion. The U.S. Food and Drug Administration barred its importation into this country in 1986. Gianna was one of those scheduled to speak. The approach to the debate taken by those supporting the drug (and therefore abortion) is instructive and all too typical of the way such discussions go.

The hall outside the hearing room looked a little like an airport terminal, Gianna thought. Armed security guards stood at the door, their eyes moving rapidly over each person as he or she passed through a metal detector, while other guards sat at desks, rummaging through purses and briefcases. A sign nearby read, "No applause, placards or demonstrations while Board is in session."

The room itself was the size of a large church sanctuary, with silver-blue velvet pews. A sloping aisle led down the middle of the hall and ended at a short, wooden wall, topped with a glass shield, that separated spectators from supervisors.

83

Settling into the front row, Gianna looked curiously across the partition. Immediately beyond it were the backs of three chairs, with three microphones on booms leaning toward them. Beyond them was a semicircle of tables with five tall, black, leather chairs facing the audience. To one side was a host of reporters, minicams, and flash equipment. A sergeant at arms stood nearby.

One by one, all five supervisors entered and seated themselves in the leather chairs. Gianna read the names on the place cards before them: Edmund Edelman, Gloria Molina, Chairman Michael Antonovich, Deane Dana, and Kenneth Hahn. The men looked grandfatherly; they didn't intimidate Gianna. But Gloria Molina was the supervisor who wanted the board to approve RU-486, and Gianna didn't feel so comfortable with her.

Gianna looked again at the agenda in her lap. The wording of Supervisor Molina's recommendation was confusing: "Support H.R. 875 (Wyden), legislation which would rescind the Food and Drug Administration's import alert on RU-486, a drug compound manufactured in France, which may be effective in treatments for a broad range of diseases and conditions . . ."

All Gianna knew or cared about was that RU-486 was a pill that could do what the abortionist had tried to do to her with an injection—end a human life.

A local pastor opened the meeting with prayer for God's wisdom and grace. "Make us a people of vision," he asked. "Give us caring. Give us understanding. Give us hearts of righteousness . . . that we will hear You and be blessed of You this day."

Then Chairman Antonovich, in the middle chair, called out three names. A man and two women in the audience rose, walked up three carpeted steps to the low wall, and pushed open a diminutive wooden door. They sat down in the three chairs facing the supervisors. *That's what I'll have to do pretty soon*, thought Gianna. *Facing that way won't be so hard, because I won't have to look at everybody. It would sure be a lot easier if I had come to sing, though.*

The first speaker leaned toward his microphone and introduced himself as Dr. Brian Connell from Loma Linda University, with degrees in medicine and law. He gave a short history of RU-486.

"Roussell-Uclaf developed this drug in 1980. Roussell is a very large, prestigious pharmaceutical company. If they were able to find a proper use for this drug outside the abortion industry, they would have done so . . ."

Then one of the women gave her name as Nancy Mullin, describing herself as a doctor and psychiatrist. She called abortion by RU-486 "a far worse ordeal than surgical abortion." At this, there was an outcry from some of the people in the audience. Gianna turned around to look at them. A motley assortment of rough-looking people filled the right side of the auditorium. Some wore T-shirts that read "Act Up."

Diana whispered to Gianna, "Act Up is a homosexual group."

"Oh," said Gianna, wondering why homosexuals cared about abortion.

Nancy Mullin was still speaking. "The abortion itself takes three days and is accompanied by heavy cramping and bleeding which can go on up to 16 days." She suggested that the county of Los Angeles might be liable for damages if the supervisors approved the drug and its use caused injury to women.

A stylishly dressed, slim blonde reached for the microphone and introduced herself as Susan Carpenter-McMillan, media spokeswoman for Right to Life. She spoke with passion as she said, "Nineteen years ago, the Supreme Court legalized abortion up through the hour of birth. That decision was brought about by a woman named Norma McCorvey, who claimed that she had been raped. That rape was a false charge. She admitted later that she never had been.

"Dr. Bernard Nathanson, the cofounder of NARAL—the

National Abortion Rights Action League—admitted that he, too, went before the Senate Judiciary Committee and lied about thousands of women dying from illegal abortions because he said later it was so important for us to legalize abortion. Well today, the pro-abortionists are at it again. As Roe versus Wade was based on a lie, so is RU-486.

"Dr. Jerome Lejeune, the famed French geneticist who discovered the Down's syndrome gene, said, 'RU-486 has one use only, and that is to destroy unborn life.'

"Dr. Nathanson said, 'The abortionist hopes to get RU-486 to be approved for a non-abortion-related purpose, so that pro-lifers will not fight it.' I urge this board to not allow the abortion pill to be brought in *regardless* of the people who will say it has nothing to do with abortion. It has *everything* to do with abortion."

As the chairman started to call the next three people forward, Carpenter-McMillan added that she had brought petitions with her from 16,000 people who were against the drug. At that, a woman shouted something from the back of the hall. Gianna felt an undercurrent of hostility in the room. It unnerved her.

Father John Moretta, pastor of Resurrection Church in East Los Angeles, read a statement from Archbishop Roger Mahony that said in part: "I urge the Board of Supervisors to reject the proposal. Clearly there is no pressing need for this action. You should be mindful of the very many citizens of the county who hold abortion to be murder. It would be an affront to all the people for the county to go out of its way to sponsor legislation that embraces so needlessly what they in conscience find abhorrent."

Marcella Malindiz spoke for Hispanic women, appealing directly to Gloria Molina: "Please don't go through with this proposal! I beg you—if necessary, on my knees. The women who will be most affected by this will be the Hispanic women, those who cannot defend themselves because of language barriers. They will be the ones used as guinea pigs.

Please don't do this to them.

"Most people are remembered for one action in their lives, and this will be the action that you will be remembered for." Her final words competed with rising objections from the pocket of hecklers in the audience. "Your name will be synonymous with death," she continued. "You will face your constituents and your God!"

Light applause broke out despite the heckling, and immediately the chairman reminded the audience, "We don't allow applause."

Then Supervisor Molina spoke. "I've made this decision many, many years ago," she said. "I've always been a pro-choice candidate." (Loud and rowdy, though brief, applause and cheers came from the homosexual contingent.) "I believe in it strongly enough to support this motion that allows for *safe, clinical, scientific* testing of a drug that will be valuable to many people who make a choice. This would be a voluntary program."

Someone from Act Up shouted "Bravo!" and there was more wild cheering.

Malindiz told Supervisor Molina brokenly, "The blood of those children will be on your hands."

The next speaker was LaVerne Tolbert, a board member of Planned Parenthood in New York City from 1975 to 1980. She spoke as a black woman. "I, too, was pro-choice," she began, "until I sat on the board and learned what the inside story was. . . .

"They do *not* have women's rights at heart. The whole motive behind the pro-abortion movement is to keep blacks and Hispanics and third-world women from having babies. It sounds ludicrous, doesn't it? I sat on the board and read documents about how we should promote abortion to keep these women from having babies.

"I am very saddened—in fact, last night I could not sleep—that RU-486 has come this far. Black women comprise only 12 percent of the population, yet over half of those women undergo abortions. Minority women are the target of the abortion movement, because we are the majority of the poor. If we do not stand up and stand against RU-486, we are going to be the victims."

The atmosphere of the room was charged with unrest and conflict, as if violence could break out at any time. To Gianna, it didn't feel safe.

The next three people called forward were a licensed psychologist, a woman who had run a crisis pregnancy center, and the president of Simon Greenleaf University. The psychologist had worked as a counselor for Planned Parenthood, and as she started to describe the psychological effects of the RU-486 pill, a murmur of disagreement around Gianna broke out into open jeering. Gianna felt she was in the middle of this, as if somehow this whole war were over her, and it confused and scared her. She was already trembling with fear and on the verge of tears—and she hadn't even gotten up to speak yet!

Terry Reisser, the woman who had run a crisis pregnancy center, claimed to have counseled hundreds of women for postabortion trauma. She read an internal memo from Planned Parenthood Federation of America to its affiliates; it confirmed "anti-choice studies and surveys" showing the incidence of postprocedural trauma in women to be as high as 91 percent of all abortion cases.

"As a counselor, I am *very* concerned about the kind of trauma that we are going to be inflicting—these women are going to be at *high* risk for postprocedural trauma because they're going to be *seeing* the fetus—an inch-long little human being with limbs."

Dr. Sam Casey, president of Simon Greenleaf University, said, "What we see is the politicization of medical research, and this board is being required to do something that it is not competent to do. This process of politicization started with AIDS research—"

Angry shouting from the audience interrupted and

attempted to drown him out.

Supervisor Hahn demanded in his gravelly voice, "Who is in the audience yelling out?"

Supervisor Molina scolded the audience for its rowdiness, and Chairman Antonovich called more names. Gianna jumped when she heard hers among them. By now her heart was pounding and her palms were damp. She felt more nervous than she ever had before.

Numbly, Gianna followed two women up the steps and through the wooden half door. They took the seats just vacated by the previous speakers. She was glad she couldn't see the hecklers behind her, but she couldn't see her mother, either, and that made her feel vulnerable and exposed. She wished Diana could have come forward with her.

Gianna scarcely heard the two women who spoke ahead of her. One was a registered nurse who cited French studies showing that "one out of a thousand women will hemorrhage severely enough to require a transfusion, and one confirmed maternal death has taken place already in France."

The other, the president of Feminists for Life of California, said, "RU-486 is not the simple morning-after pill that we've been promised. It's lethal to children in the womb and dangerous to women. Please don't allow this chemical warfare against women and their children."

Those two women seemed to have taken no time at all, and suddenly Gianna found herself speaking into the microphone pointed at her. She heard her voice amplified and wondered if it sounded as scared as she felt. Her heart thudding, she began, "My name is Gianna Jessen, and I'm 14 years old." She took a deep, shaky breath. "My biological mother chose to have a saline abortion in her third trimester. She was seven months along. But I survived—only by the grace of God, I believe."

There was hooting from the audience, jeers, and cries of what sounded like "Poor baby!"

Why doesn't somebody make those people stop? Gianna

wondered. Inside, she was terrified, but she kept talking as steadily as she could. "After spending about three and a half months in—"

Behind her, from the sea of Act Up T-shirts, a man made a loud sobbing sound, or was it a groan? Gianna's heart lurched. Was someone touched by her story? No, the sound was mocking her. She kept going. "—in the hospital, I was—"

There it was again. A man was pretending to sob. Something within her said, *He's lying, just to get you to break down.* "I was placed . . . placed"— her voice wavered—"in a foster home—"

Supervisor Hahn interrupted abruptly. "What noise do I hear?" he demanded.

Gianna stopped talking, but the crying sounds only got louder. Starting at the front of the hearing room, they were picked up by other pro-abortionists, and the auditorium was soon full of fake sobbing sounds and an undercurrent of people whispering.

It was too much for Gianna. She burst into tears.

"Just relax, Gianna," the chairman said encouragingly.

Supervisor Hahn instructed an aide sharply, "Give her some water."

Meanwhile, Diana had bolted from her seat and raced to her daughter's side. *How can they allow heckling like this in a supervisors' meeting?* she wondered. *Do those Act Up people really think they can win a debate by intimidating and scaring a teenage girl?* At least the hearing room in Alabama had been controlled. There were pro-abortion people there, too, but they hadn't interrupted the proceedings. She squatted down next to Gianna, who was sobbing brokenheartedly, and put her arms around her.

"Okay?" asked the chairman.

"Okay," repeated Gianna, trying to laugh at herself.

Diana offered to escort her out, but Gianna shook her head. Her voice came out determinedly, between gasps. "I am going to speak . . . exactly . . . what . . . is on my mind! I am

14 years old . . . and . . . I . . . am sitting . . . in front of you . . . doing . . . the best that I c-ca-can . . . to tell you . . . my story . . . all right? I'm . . . sorry. I'm trying . . . to pull myself together . . . okay? And I want to tell you the story."

Why are the people in the audience so angry at me? she thought. *I haven't done anything to them. I'm just giving the facts about the way I came into the world. They're treating me as if I did something bad by surviving an abortion!*

She paused and tried to get her breath. She even laughed a little. She continued, with dry sobs and sniffs punctuating her sentences like little hiccups. "Like I said, my . . . biological mother . . . was 17, and she had . . . an abortion in her third trimester, but I survived. When I was placed in a foster home, I was diagnosed with cerebral palsy as a result . . . of . . . the saline ab-abortion.

"At the beginning of this hearing, there was a prayer, and it was asked unto God for a vision and His blessing. But let me say, do you think by letting RU-486 come into Los Angeles, do you think God is happy about that? Do you think He likes . . . watching His children die?" She was starting to cry again. "I mean, you're killing someone's best friend, maybe your grandchild or *my* best friend or something. How can you stand by and let that happen?

"So I'm just here . . . to tell you . . . I'm telling you not to vote and let it come in here, because it's just going to do more damage than it does good. That's all I have to say. Thank you."

"Thank you, Gianna," said the chairman quietly.

Diana helped Gianna stand and walked her through the door, down the steps, and up the aisle, while reporters and photographers scrambled to follow. The unruly mob on one side of the room jeered and booed as they left, calling out, "Exploiting a poor little child!"

Across the room, Gianna caught the blazing eyes of a man in a suit, and she knew it was the man who had started the crying noises. He slipped out the door before she did.

Diana and Gianna walked outside, past the sign about no applause or demonstrations during board sessions, with Gianna still sobbing. The man in the suit was waiting for them. As Gianna leaned helplessly against a wall, he glared at her, his eyes cutting through her.

"Oh, yeah!" he jeered. "Bring the press around!"

Why, why does he hate me? Gianna wondered. *What have I done?*

Diana was thinking, *Won't these pro-choice people let anyone who disagrees with them have a fair hearing?*

Nothing about Gianna was shown on TV. The next day, the *Los Angeles Times* referred to Gianna only obliquely: "The Los Angeles County Board of Supervisors, after an emotional debate pitting opponents of abortion against abortion-rights activists, endorsed congressional legislation on Tuesday that would allow importation of the French abortion pill RU-486." The motion passed 4-1, with Mike Antonovich casting the lone dissenting vote.

Afterward, Supervisor Antonovich wrote Gianna a letter, saying in part, "I . . . commend you on your courageous remarks. You touched many hearts and made people question their beliefs.

"While we were not successful in our efforts, I know that our Lord will recognize you and all of those who are fighting for the sanctity of life."

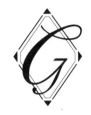

Braving
the Death-
Scorts

chapter 10

Sitting alone on the top step of Midtown Hospital, her back against its metal doors, Gianna shivered. It was only 5:00 in the morning, but she wasn't cold, not here in Atlanta in late July 1991. She was scared, "scared out of my boots," as she would later tell a reporter from the Christian girls' magazine *Brio*.

Gianna had volunteered, along with 11 other kids ages eight to 16, to try to shut down, at least for a day, this three-story, 60,000-square-foot building dedicated solely to abortion.

What am I doing here? thought Gianna. *Jessi and I didn't come to Atlanta to get involved in something like this! We could get ourselves arrested!* She remembered Thursday night, when she had sung and spoken at the Youth for America rally that kicked off the four-day second annual National Youth Rescue. *That's why I came, to tell my story and sing. But I do want to take a stand for the unborn.*

After her time on stage Thursday night, 15-year-old Steven Rella had spoken. He talked about rescues—direct, physical attempts to prevent abortions—and he described those he had personally participated in, resulting in 150 arrests.

Gianna agreed that stopping abortions was important, but when Steven encouraged the youthful audience to join him on Friday and Saturday, she shrank back. The thought of once again having to come into contact with people who believed in a woman's right to abort a baby made her stomach tighten and her throat go dry.

The next night, Gianna, Diana, and Jessi sat curiously

through a second rally, this one led by 12-year-old Laurel Foreman. They listened as young people described enthusiastically how they had spent the day scaling fences, blocking driveways, and resisting the physical and psychological attacks of "pro-aborts" at the Northside Women's Center in nearby Chamblee. Several of the rescuers said the persecution they had experienced made them feel closer to Christ.

Joseph Foreman, Laurel's father, gave the keynote speech at the rally. Then Laurel offered the same invitation Steven had given: "Join us tomorrow morning."

"Let's just meet with them and see what they're going to do," suggested Jessi. They stayed up till 1:30 in the morning talking about it, "really hyper and excited," as Jessi put it. When they finally got to sleep, it seemed just minutes before Diana was shaking Gianna awake.

"If you guys are going, you have half an hour," she said. It wasn't even light yet. Gianna pulled on a T-shirt with a big, red sign reading "STOP Abortion" on it, and the two of them joined the group going to the rescue. They remembered not to eat or drink anything so they wouldn't need to go to the bathroom.

Steven and Laurel were already there, and so were others, including Laurel's eight-year-old brother, Josh, a veteran rescuer. There was also a 16-year-old girl with long, dark hair, bangs, and freckles. Her name was Jenny Morson. Jenny, Gianna found out, headed up Youth for America in Maryland.

Steven greeted them. "Our target is Midtown Hospital," he said. "All they do there are abortions. There are 12 of us and nine ways to get in. We'll split up into pairs and block the doors the best we can. What the pro-aborts usually do is gang together and attack one door at a time, trying to break through. If they can't break through, they'll run to the next one."

Then Laurel prayed. She asked God naively to make them as heavy as boulders.

Midtown Hospital was "a big, scary building—an ugly,

brick thing, all dirty and stuff," according to Jessi. The hospital was already open when the teenagers arrived. Jessi and Gianna were assigned one of the big, metal doors. The first person who tried to open it was a man on the *inside* wanting to get *out*.

Two designated escorts—volunteers determined to get the mothers into the building ("death-scorts," the rescuers called them)—stood at the entrance. They were both smoking, and they both flicked their ashes on the girls. Gianna started to talk to one of them, telling her story and then talking about Jesus.

The woman stopped her abruptly with "How do you know Jesus wasn't a woman?"

At another door, two of the girls were trying to keep out a young woman coming for an abortion with her boyfriend. Jessi ran to help them, and Gianna suddenly found herself alone. *It's my first rescue,* she thought. *Where is everybody?* She felt small, vulnerable, and shaky. "Lord, be with me!" she prayed. "Please help me!"

She heard a commotion around the corner. Angry women were shouting and pounding on doors, and men's voices were ordering the rescuers to move. She heard the faint strains of "Amazing grace, how sweet the sound that saved a wretch like me . . ." Superimposed on it, to the same tune, were other, determined voices singing, "Pro-choice! Pro-choice! Pro-choice! Pro-choice!"

How dumb! thought Gianna. *How rude!* Besides fear, she felt anger. She looked up. A security guard, legs spread and arms behind his back, stood facing her. She caught his eye and tried to talk to him.

"Your clinic does late-term abortions, doesn't it?" she said.

"No," he replied.

"I've heard that they do. I've heard that they don't do anything but abortions here and that many of them are late-term."

"They might do a few."

"My birth mother aborted me," said Gianna softly, keeping her eyes on his. "She was seven months pregnant. But I survived."

The guard just stood there. His eyes were troubled now. Gianna could see questions in them—doubts and uneasiness.

"I have cerebral palsy because of the abortion."

The guard never said another word.

Gianna tried singing to give herself courage. Suddenly the voices got louder, and with them were scuffling noises and the sound of running feet. From around the corner came a mob of people, full tilt, shouting obscenities and making gestures: pregnant women and their boyfriends, guards, hospital personnel, escorts.

"Lord Jesus, be with me. Lord Jesus, please help me. Please keep me safe," Gianna prayed. She stared at the people with terrified eyes, her heart pounding. Within her, prayers ran together in a torrent. She sang with all her might, but her quavering voice was scarcely audible over the chaos. She wondered if anyone could hear her.

"Get away from the door!" someone shouted. At the next door, hands and knees tried to shove Jenny out of the way. The death-scorts were kicking and beating her—and screaming "Assault!" although she wasn't retaliating.

Gianna's teeth were chattering, but she continued singing about God's love.

"We don't care about you or your God!" a woman in the back of the crowd yelled at her. "You're being brainwashed!"

You're the ones being brainwashed, thought Gianna. She had never felt so surrounded by evil as she did now. It was a force almost physical. She could practically visualize demons swirling about her, looking for points of weakness.

From a grassy embankment at the rear of the clinic, Diana sat with another parent, watching over their children and praying. Apprehension turned to peace as she felt God's protective arms around her daughter.

Security guards were struggling with all their might at the clinic doors, but they weren't budging. *As heavy as boulders,* Gianna remembered. To her relief, her terror moderated a bit.

God and Satan are battling it out, she thought, *and I'm right in the middle of it!* She had a surge of confidence. *God is protecting us. I can be a witness for the Lord.*

Gianna called out to one pregnant woman, "Please don't abort your child like my mom did to me." The woman went on into the clinic, but apparently Gianna's words stayed with her, because soon she came out again to announce she had decided not to abort the child after all.

Police cars drove up and assembled in a parking lot across the street. Two officers with batons in hand walked the perimeter of the building, asking the determined teens if this was their first rescue. "No?" they said. "Well, how about that. They're all a bunch of veterans!"

The presence of a CNN camera crew kept the police at a distance, as brutality claims had recently been rocking the local department. Gianna gave CNN reporters a courteous interview, and a cameraman encouraged her.

Meanwhile, eight-year-old Josh was having a standoff with pro-aborts at the front door of the clinic. His small body pressed the door tightly, but a violent shove from inside crushed him between the glass door, the brick wall, and the iron railing. His cherubic face winced with pain, and he struggled to keep from crying as one eye began to swell and a cheek to discolor.

There were fewer women arriving now. As one car holding two women pulled into the parking lot, Gianna left the hospital door to walk up and speak to the driver.

"Your baby is alive!" she said, reaching into the car to pat her stomach. "Don't—"

"I'm not pregnant!" snapped the driver. She jerked her head toward the passenger in the front seat. "*She* is!"

The two women parked and got out. They made it to the door before the rescuers did and slipped inside.

Meanwhile, Jenny was running up the sidewalk toward an approaching woman. "Please don't kill your baby!" she pleaded.

The woman's answer carried all the way down the street: "I'm not fertile!"

Someone was coming out of the hospital. Gianna turned and saw the two women she had spoken to in the car. They came up to her, and the one who was pregnant said, "I've changed my mind."

"Praise the Lord!" Gianna said. She wasn't cold or scared anymore. She was overflowing with joy.

By 8:15 that morning, the women with appointments had stopped coming in. At least for a few hours, 12 kids shut down the second-largest abortion facility in Atlanta. And not one of them had been arrested.

Weeks later, Gianna was describing her experience at the rescue to a congregation in California. "I wasn't arrested at the first clinic," she told them, "so we went to another clinic." The audience laughed, and Gianna, realizing how that had come out, laughed with them. "I mean, our *time* was over at that clinic."

Their next target was the Women's Health Clinic, located in a medical building. The teens marched in the front door, up one flight of stairs, and down the hall to the wooden door at the end. There was only one door to guard this time. The little group sat down with their backs to it. Then they prayed and sang.

Before long, a woman inside forced open the door and introduced herself as the manager of the clinic. The young people kept singing, "Mr. Policeman, tell me why/unborn babies have to die./Keep your eyes on the prize./Hold on!"

"Now, children," the manager said sweetly, "do you know what you're doing here?"

One of them interrupted the song to answer her, "Yes, ma'am, we do."

"Well, do you know it's against the law?"

"Yes, ma'am." They sang louder.

"If you don't move, I'll have to call the police, honey."

"Ma'am, we're not moving."

She shook her head and said, as if to herself, "Oh, they're just so young to be doing this!" and then to them, "I'll give you one last chance. Leave or I'll call the police!"

"We're staying here."

"So she calls the police," Gianna told the author afterward, on the landing of her home in San Clemente. "They bring in about 20 police officers—not literally, but I mean, just so many! For teenagers! I mean, we're *not* that *heavy*.

"This big, husky man goes, 'Do you *know* what you're doing?'

"We go, 'Yes, we do.' And I go, 'But do *you* know why we're here? We're doing this to save the unborn babies.'

" 'You have no right to be here. It's against the law.'

" 'There's a higher law.'

" 'You can't prove that.'

" 'And we believe that God's here.'

"And he said, 'There is no god here.'

"And we said, 'Excuse me, sir—yes, there is!'

"All this time I'm just crying, 'cause it's my first day of rescuing, and I'm thinking, *What am I going to do?*

"We pleaded with them not to arrest us so we could continue to protect children. Jenny told one of them, 'It's awful to be aborted.'

"He said, 'You don't know what it's like to be aborted,' and Jenny said, 'But Gianna does.' When I told my story, he had nothing to say.

"Then he put me under arrest. He looks at me and he goes, 'I'll help you up.' So he pulls me up, and I decided to walk instead of going limp. I didn't want to get hurt because I already have a disability. Jessi walked, too. He shoved us in the police car. Jenny went limp and had to be carried. She goes, 'Don't throw me on her!' meaning me, you know, but they threw her on top of me anyway.

"In the police car, I'm just thinking, *Omigosh, I can't believe I'm here*. But at the same time I'm praying, 'Thank You, Lord! I'm glad I'm here. I don't want to be hurt or anything, so please protect me.'"

The rescuers were driven to the police station and booked for disorderly conduct. Gianna showed the author her wrinkled arrest citation, #903639: "Blocked entrance to surgical center and refused to leave."

"We sat there, all of us, for four hours. Josh's face was turning black and blue. They filled out *all* these forms, and then they took us to juvenile hall. One officer goes, 'You're going to be put in with murderers, and you'll be in there forever, and this will be on your record, and you'll never be a lawyer, you'll never be a doctor.'"

But at juvenile hall, they were released into the custody of their parents, and the charges were dropped.

At that evening's victory celebration, the excited young people discussed their experiences. "The more you rescue, the more you get called Jesus freaks," Gianna said. "It's a perfect example of what it says in the Bible, that Christians will be hated."

Apart from a local paper, which ran a small article on a back page about juveniles being arrested for blocking the doors of Northside Women's Center, the media ignored the entire series of youth rescues.

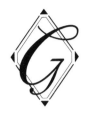

A
Ministry
Takes
Off

chapter 11

By autumn 1991, Gianna was traveling and speaking full-time: Northern California, Oregon, Washington, New York City, Sioux Falls. She helped launch a new radio station in Phoenix. She made public-service announcements on television for a pro-life campaign in Boston. She was home so infrequently that she joked about attending "airplane school."

On a September evening, Gianna was at Mayfair Community Church in Lakewood, California. Her program that night was typical of how she related to audiences as her fledgling singing and speaking ministry took flight.

As she was introduced, Gianna came to the microphone at the foot of the platform steps and took it off its stand. She wore a black jacket and shorts, and she had woven two little braids on one side of her head and combed out her bangs.

"You'll have to excuse me," she told the audience informally. "I don't have any shoes on because if I keep my shoes on, I'll lose my balance, and one minute you'll see me standing up, and the next minute you'll see me on the floor."

It wasn't only her balance that was problematic that evening. She started to speak but couldn't seem to express herself. "First I'd like to open . . . uh, by singing . . . by just kind of . . . uh, well, I'm gonna sing this song, and I want you to . . . I want you to . . . sing it after me, sing it with me."

Gianna looked relieved to have the sentence out, and the audience smiled back at her sympathetically. Together they sang "Awesome God," and as their voices blended, Gianna felt the room really was filled with His wisdom, power, and love. Her face beamed with excitement.

She had sung without a hitch. Sitting in the front row, Diana let herself relax.

"This next song really means a lot to me because it talks about, you know, us and God. It's saying, 'Who am I, Jesus, that You would call me by name?' He just loves us so much, He . . . He called us to . . . to serve Him, and to . . . to . . ." Gianna was stumbling over her words again. This time she confronted her difficulty head-on.

"You'll have to excuse me," she told the crowd again. "See, sometimes I have what I want to say in my head, but it's hard for me to get it out. So be patient with me."

She sang Margaret Becker's "Who Am I?" which speaks humbly of God's deep love for us. It was especially plaintive in her sweet soprano.

Then she walked up to the platform, and it was obvious she was still feeling vulnerable. "I hope I don't fall going up these steps . . . I made it. Hallelujah! Sometimes I'll be walking up steps, and I'll just fall right over. Anyway—" This time trying to get the right words out was even worse. "Uh . . . we . . . some . . . I . . . uh . . ."

In her characteristically candid way, Gianna stopped again and admitted "I just need to pray right now," and she did, out loud. "Heavenly Father, give me all the words to say, and calm my nerves." When she finished, she sighed and said, "Ahh, that always helps!"

As she went on to describe her next song, the awkwardness fell away from her, and the audience was drawn to what she was saying rather than to how she was saying it. "There are times in our lives when you can just feel the spiritual warfare. Like when you're rescuing. There are people who say, 'What you stand for is stupid. You're just an *idiot!*'

"And you've got other people saying, 'Come on, you can do it.' You've got God over here, too, saying, 'Oh, I love what you're doing! You're standing for Me. You're standing in the fire.' That's what my next song is about. Listen to the words."

Every day I hear it—evil is abroad
making even children enemies of God.
Yet somehow I always find above the crowd
other voices pleading, crying truth aloud.
And I don't know your name,
But I think I see your face.
I see you standing in the fire,
standing on the Word.

I SEE YOU STANDING by Twila Paris
Used by permission.

As the last notes and the applause quieted, Gianna said, "You may have heard it, but I'm going to tell you my story now. Pray that I don't just go 'um, um, um.'" There was no audible response, but she knew she was being upheld by prayer.

After the usual summary of her birth mother's abortion, she spoke about the cerebral palsy responsible for the problems that had become obvious to the audience that evening. "I have to do physical therapy," she told them. "I don't always like to sit down and do my stretches—not that it hurts, but it takes too much time.

"But the thing that is difficult is like, in school you get treated totally differently if you have a disability—*totally* differently—and I don't think a person can fully understand how you get treated unless you have a disability. It's like you're a totally different *being.*

"I was in school, and I had a real rough time because everybody wanted to be cool, and you weren't cool if you hung out with a person with a disability. I would make a friend in school, and the relationship was fine for a while. Then they'd disappear. I thought that was pretty crummy, you know?"

She described how the teachers had offered to provide her with "book buddies."

"They were trying to be real helpful, but being in the seventh and eighth grade, you don't want someone walking around going, 'Okay, let me take your bag' or 'I'll help you with this.' You don't want that. You say, 'Get out of here, I can do it on my own!' You know? I don't need help all the time. I mean, it would get on your nerves after a while. So that didn't work out too well.

"We went to the school psychologist and the principal, and I said, 'I want to be home schooled now,' and I could *not believe* these words came out of his mouth. He sat there and looked my mom and me in the face, and he said, 'We can get some people to hang out with you. We can get you some volunteer friends.' That just ate me up. I was just sitting there going, *Gianna, control yourself! Control yourself!* I was ready to stand up and go *pow!*" She made a punching motion with her right fist. "I was!

"Can you imagine someone staring you *right in the eye* saying 'We can get you some volunteer friends'? It's like, 'I'll give them an *A* to hang out with you!' So I bailed—er, I left the school—and I've been home schooled ever since. So that's cool.

"That part of having cerebral palsy is very difficult. Otherwise, I don't even know I have it. It's like it's not even there.

"Being an abortion survivor is kind of difficult, too. I have some fears. People are fighting over abortion. We know there's life inside the womb, but there's a whole bunch of people out there who couldn't care less, who are not informed. And it's scary when you go out and speak. Most of the time, there's someone in the audience that believes in abortion, and here you're going, 'O, Lord!' You don't know what's going to happen from one minute to the next. Not that I'm ever in any danger, but it's a scary thought for me, you know what I'm saying? I have to rely on God every step of the way.

"He's my strength every day. That's what my next song is about. Feel free to sing along. It's just a praise song. If you listen to these words, it's almost identical to my life, because there are some days I just say, 'Lord, I can't get through this day,' and He says, 'Yes, you can! Just get up and go out there, and I'll be with you.' " Then she closed singing these words:

I open my eyes to the sound
of the morning news
And wish for ten more minutes
left to sleep.
And as I get into the shower,
the thoughts of facing one more day
Overwhelm me, and I begin to weep.
And I've never felt like I've needed
Your help so bad. . . .
Every day I look to You to be
the strength of my life.
You're the hope I hold onto.
Be the strength of my life.
When I learn to know my weakness,
I understand Your strength. . . .
Be the strength of my life,
the strength of my life,
Be the strength of my life today.

STRENGTH OF MY LIFE by Leslie Phillips
Used by permission.

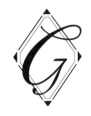

National TV
and the
Unknown
Viewer

chapter 12

Half a continent away, Gianna's birth mother was now living in Indiana. *This state is beautiful in the fall*, Tina thought, gazing out her window. *Southern California weather doesn't get like this till January.* This afternoon the leaves were crisp, brown, and orange, and the air was cool, inviting her to go out. The 31-year-old woman was bored, but she stayed inside.

She and her husband had moved to Indiana a year before to be near his dying mother. After her death, they rented an apartment in her husband's hometown, Fortville. They had brought one of Tina's brothers with them, and he was sitting at the kitchen table now, idly flicking through the channels on their portable TV.

At 1:00 in the afternoon, there wasn't much on. Soaps. Reruns. A talk show. He paused at the talk show, and when Tina glanced at the set, her breath caught. On the screen was a young teenager, a perky-looking little thing with wavy, blonde hair cascading from where it was gathered by a white bow on top of her head. Tina caught only a few words before her brother switched to another channel.

"Whoa! Turn back!" Tina cried. "That's my daughter!"

"Oh, I'm sure," he responded.

"She is! I know she is! She's got my face, my eyes! She's the same age as Giana [she had no way of knowing the pronunciation and spelling had been changed], and it says she was aborted. Turn back!"

Her brother shrugged and said, "You're full of it."

"Turn it *back*."

He checked a few other channels first, apparently decided there was nothing else worth watching, and flipped back to the talk show.

Maury Povich, the host and a personable man, had just said something to Gianna, and the teenager was giggling. Tina couldn't absorb what they were saying. She just stared hungrily at the set. Gianna wore a light-colored, floral-print dress with a wide collar and a petticoat of white lace, over white tights. *How beautiful she is!* Tina marveled. *I was so sure I would never see her again.*

Memories were flooding back. The precious, squalling baby cupped in her hands. Awe at the life contained in such a minute package. Almost physical guilt because she had almost taken that life. Anger that people who knew better had told her it wasn't wrong.

"That's my daughter!" she said again, not realizing she had spoken aloud.

"Oh, I'm sure," her brother repeated scathingly, but she didn't hear him.

"What were you told about being given up?" Povich was asking. He seemed warm and sympathetic.

Tina leaned forward, tense. *Giana's talking about me!*

"I was told that my biological mother was very, very young—only 17—and that she wasn't able to take care of me at that time, so she had to give me up to people that could give me a loving home."

In Indiana, tears ran unheeded down Tina's face.

"When were you told all this? How old were you?"

Gianna hesitated. "When was I told that I was aborted or that I was given up?"

"Both."

"I was told that I was given up from the time I was very, very small. In my foster home, I knew."

"When did you find out the real story about the abortion attempt?"

"When I was 12 years old. It was on Christmas Day. We

were making Christmas dinner. I said, 'Mom, why do I have this disability? Why do I have cerebral palsy?'

"I had asked her that I don't know how many times. But for the first time, she said, 'Do you really want to know why?' and I said, 'Yes, I do,' and she said, 'You'd better sit down' and I said, 'No, that's okay, I'll stand up.' And she said, 'Well, your mother was seven months pregnant, and she— she—' As soon as the words were about to come out, I filled in the words. I said, 'I was aborted, right?'

"Now, don't tell me how I knew, because I did not know for 12 years, but at that moment—"

Povich interrupted her with amazement. "You seem to know everything!" he said. "You seem to know everything, Gianna! I mean, you're about going on 35 or 40!" Everyone was laughing now. "I can't believe this!"

Still wearing a big grin, Gianna went on, "But at that moment, I feel—this is the way I really feel—God gave me that. He told me at that right moment so that I could accept it and it just wouldn't be a big *boom* for me."

"How did you react?"

"I said, 'Okay. Fine.' "

Diana, who was on the program with Gianna, added, "She said, 'Well, at least I have cerebral palsy for a unique reason. At least it's interesting.' "

In Indiana, Tina's heart was racing. *Giana, I want to tell you how it was, how sorry I am! If I contact the station, could I talk to you? Would you want to hear from me? Or would I just hurt you more than I already have?*

"What is the connection between the abortion and cerebral palsy?" Povich was asking Diana. "I don't quite understand."

"Gulping the saline solution in the womb—the saline burns. Lack of oxygen—"

"So if someone by chance survives, there is going to be this result?"

Diana and Gianna glanced at each other. "Well," said

Diana, "she's pretty lucky." Gianna nodded. "With other ones, it's usually more severe."

Gianna spoke up cheerfully. "Like she said, the baby is burned in the womb, and I have absolutely no burns on me!"

Diana added, "We know of two others, and they have some scarring."

"Why don't you stand up for a second!" Povich ordered Gianna, and as she did, "This is somebody who could not walk, could not crawl—"

Applause drowned out the end of his sentence. He rose from his chair and stepped beside her, putting an arm around her shoulders and facing the audience. He looked down at her; Gianna barely came to his shoulder.

"You're still going through some procedures. You're wearing a cast. Any more surgeries?"

Gianna clasped her hands together and looked imploringly up into his face, shrinking back into his embrace. But there was a broad smile on her face. "Hopefully not!" she exclaimed fervently. The ingenuousness of her reply and the sparkle in her eye were captivating. Povich gave her a hug.

Although the shock of seeing her daughter was so intense it was almost unbearable, the woman watching could not tear her eyes away. *Am I imagining all this?* she asked herself. *Is this just another dream? If I look away, will it all disappear?*

After a commercial break, people in the audience asked questions. There were three, all for Marilyn Miller, an abortion survivor interviewed before Gianna. And then a woman asked Gianna a question that made the woman watching in Indiana put a hand to her heart, her breath suspended: "Would you ever like to meet your real mom?"

Yes, Giana, would you? Would you?

Tina's hazel eyes were riveted on Gianna as the girl said candidly, "I don't feel like I would at this point, because I have my family. My mom's sitting right here. It's not that I am mad at my biological mother at all. I forgive her totally for what she did."

"Aww," went the audience, but the woman watching didn't hear any more. Her mind kept repeating, *"Would you ever like to meet your real mom?"* *"I don't feel like I would at this point. I have my family."*

She turned off the set and tried to turn off the disappointment flooding her. *She said no. She said she doesn't want to meet me. I'd better stay away.*

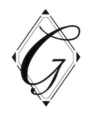

"That's What God Wants Me to Do"

chapter 13

Questions about Gianna's attitude toward her biological mother come up all the time—so often that Gianna once told an audience, "My *favorite* question is about my biological *father*, because hardly anyone ever asks it."

In interview after interview, Gianna said, "I forgive my biological mother for what she did. I'm not mad at her at all. She probably had no hope and no place else to turn, and she was only 17. But even if she was 30, 35, or 40, I would still want to forgive her, because that's what God wants me to do."

The British magazine *HELLO!*, which translated back into English her comments published in *¡HOLA!* put some big words in Gianna's mouth, but the thought was certainly hers: "If I had the chance of changing my past, I wouldn't do it, because I've completely assimilated it. I'm happy with my destiny and with what life has given me."

Sometimes she speaks of what meeting might do to her and her birth mother: "She may still be hurting, and I'm not ready for that. I don't know if I will ever be ready to meet her."

Gianna was *Brio's* cover girl in April 1992. "What if I walked up to her house and her husband answered the door?" she asked in that interview. "What would I say? 'Hi! I'm your wife's biological daughter'? That could really mess up her family."

In June, the *Globe* published an interview in which Gianna said, "I have forgiven my birth mother but I never

121

want to meet her or even to know who she is. I can only hope that she has straightened her life out."

Occasionally someone will ask Gianna how she feels about the doctor who aborted her. That doctor claims that he "started with nothing." Six months after aborting Gianna, according to an article titled "Abortion Clinic Doctor: 'Applying Principles of Good Business' " in the Orange County section of the *Los Angeles Times*, he was "a millionaire several times over."

With the income from clinics all over Southern California, "he flies between his various enterprises in his own plane, which is based at Long Beach Airport near his beachfront apartment.

"He owns a 165-acre ranch stocked with quarter horses .... He has dealings in land and cattle."

The doctor admitted in print that he runs an assembly line and prides himself on his ability to perform an abortion in under five minutes, thus eliminating "needless patient-physician contact."

As a result, he and his staff at one hospital in California did 250,000 abortions in ten years—17,000 during the year before abortion was legalized in the rest of the country. His nearest competitor was doing 6,000.

What kind of man is he? Polite, candid, and articulate, he could pass for a professor. He is politically conservative, although in 1985, the state Republican Party reportedly returned his $10,000 contribution because of its anti-abortion stand.

The doctor used to speak to church groups when invited, even though his clinics and his home, protected by 16 security guards, are regularly picketed by pro-life people. He does not respond to their shouts of "Murderer!"

Although he considers himself "one of the experts at doing second-trimester abortions," he told the congregation of a church in 1984, "I struggle with their morality. You may say there's no difference at all between an embryo 15 seconds after it's fertilized and a fetus at 24 weeks' gestation. I can't go for that. I think there's a vast difference, a vast difference in every way.

"I have great difficulty with Roe v. Wade on second-trimester abortions. I do them and do them quite commonly. It's been in the last two or three years one of the real trying questions of my own personal existence. I really feel that the court . . . erred when they made that judgment."

But by November 8, 1992, doing late abortions apparently no longer troubled this doctor. He was still doing them, and he told the *Press-Enterprise* in Riverside, California, "If someone has trouble with abortion, that is something they have to sort out on their own. I have sorted it out on my own."

As Gianna would later tell the reporter from *Brio* magazine, "I guess some people would think that I'd actually hate [the abortionist]. But I don't. I don't know how I'd react if he was sitting right here. But I think he's a pretty sick man, and I can't sit here and not forgive him. I believe that God would forgive him if he repented, so I really feel that I can forgive him."

On October 23, 1991, Gianna and Diana were guests on KSCB-TV in Sioux Falls, South Dakota. Barbara Elkjer, who hosted the special interview, chose to focus on Gianna's attitude toward her disability and the abortion that doctors told Diana was responsible for it.

As soon as the greetings and introductions were over, Elkjer commented to Gianna, "You're not bitter and resentful."

"I can't be angry or bitter—I can't," said Gianna earnestly. "First, because I'm a Christian. We can't walk around being mad at everything."

"Why not?" asked Elkjer. "A lot of people feel that they've been done wrong and have every *right* to be angry."

Gianna amended her remarks. "I mean, you can be angry, but what matters is what you do with that anger. You can turn it into sin. Or you can turn it over to the Lord."

"How did you keep from bitterness? Were there times when you were tempted to hate the world?"

"I've never really been mad at the world. I'm not the type of person that can stay angry very long. I can't be mad at my birth mother, because a person that has an abortion is a person without hope."

"And you have hope?"

"Yes, I have hope in Jesus and a family that loves me. I love my life. It's great!"

Elkjer smiled at her enthusiasm. "How did the Lord teach you to forgive? You spoke last night at the Alpha Center Banquet about being rejected in junior high for your disability. How did you learn to forgive? I see in you a victorious overcoming."

"You've just gotta take it to the Lord. That's all I can say. I remember days when I would just come home and just cry and cry and cry and get it all out. I'd sit there and cry in Mom's arms and say, 'Mom, I can't handle this! This is too much! Every time I go to school, I'm stared at, I'm unaccepted, I'm treated differently. It's not fun. I don't enjoy myself, and you're supposed to enjoy yourself in school. You're supposed to have friends and just grow up and have a good time!'"

Elkjer put in, "It's supposed to be the time of your life."

"Junior high is difficult anyway, and when you have a disability, it makes it all the harder."

"So you're saying it's okay to have those feelings. A lot of people have a very false idea that you're not supposed to feel hurt—"

"Like you're supposed to keep it inside—"

"That you're a Christian, so you don't get hurt, you don't let these wounds affect you when people are nasty to you. But you did. You went home and cried."

Elkjer turned to Diana and asked how she had helped Gianna deal with those hurts. Diana explained that she had taught Gianna to confront people's questions head-on, beginning when Gianna was young. She also described Gianna's persistence in trying new things and being included in all the activities other kids were doing.

One month after the Maury Povich program that Gianna's biological mother watched, Gianna and Diana were interviewed on "Table Talk." The nationally syndicated Christian radio program features host Rich Buhler. Gianna, who is always looking for father figures anyway, took to Buhler right away.

"He's one of those men that I just love because they have a heart for God—a real tender heart—and they practice what they preach," she confided to a reporter.

Buhler is from Arizona and looks as if he might be a country singer. With his blond beard and open-necked shirts, you'd never guess he's an ordained minister.

Buhler has a soft heart when it comes to children—he has seven of his own—and especially when it comes to adopted children, since he's one himself. He cares about all those affected by abortion and has interviewed women all along the spectrum of life versus choice. When Operation Rescue came to Los Angeles to block clinic doors, he went to the front lines for a firsthand account. He ended up so impressed by the sanity and courage of the rescuers that he eventually joined them for a rescue and got arrested.

After the interview, Diana talked to Buhler privately. As Gianna's speaking and singing schedule expanded, taking her all over the country, one concern had been nagging at Diana. Somewhere out there was the woman who had given birth to Gianna. But where? Would she show up at one of Gianna's concerts, maybe cause a scene? What if she was some kind of crazy person? Diana confided all this to Buhler. "How would it affect Gianna to have a stranger confront her somewhere and say, 'I'm your mother'? If I just knew the city she lived in, I could at least prepare Gianna and head off a crisis. I've tried to trace her, but I've run into a dead end."

"I have a friend who's a private investigator," said Buhler. "Let me see what he can do."

When he got home, Buhler called Pat Rutherford, founder and director of WorldWide Tracers in San Clemente. "Pat," he said, "I've got a case for you. It's tugging at my heart. A woman adopted a little girl who was aborted and survived. She's looking for the birth mother, and she's going to be calling you."

Rutherford, who calls Buhler "the finest Christian I have ever met," would do just about anything for him. So he agreed, as a favor, to find Gianna Jessen's birth mother.

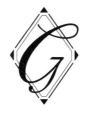

Answering
the
Skeptics

On October 27, 1991, the *New York Times* ran a cynical front-page article contrasting Gianna with another teenage girl named Becky Bell:
"In Debate on Abortion, 2 Girls Make It Real."

Said the *Times:* "Gianna Jessen, the girl who lived when she was supposed to die, and Becky Bell, the girl who died when she was supposed to live, have become the symbols of the nation's bitter debate over abortion—poster girls whose stories are being shrewdly marketed by their supporters to keep passions high.

"To sell anything in America, even an idea, it helps to have a human face and story to make it real.

"For anti-abortion groups, who are trying to make the case that each of the 1.6 million abortions performed in this country each year kills a living being, the face is that of Gianna Jessen. The California teen-ager's mother tried a saline abortion 14 years ago, and it left Gianna with cerebral palsy, but did not kill her. . . .

"For abortion-rights groups trying to show the hardships women suffer when abortion is restricted, the face is that of Becky Bell, a 17-year-old Indianapolis girl who died in 1988 from a botched abortion because she was afraid to get her parents' consent, as the state law required. Since Becky's death, her parents, Karen and Bill, have traveled to 23 states to testify or lobby against parental notification laws."

The article was lengthy and was widely reprinted. In it, some doubt was cast on the likelihood of Gianna's really having been aborted:

"Abortion-rights advocates . . . stress that it is impossible for them to verify that Gianna was aborted because her birth certificate and other records are confidential."

It wasn't the first time. On October 5, 1991, the *Washington Times* quoted Diana's claim that "one out of every 400 babies aborted by saline abortion is born alive" and went on to say, "Susan Shermer, National Abortion Federation, could not confirm Mrs. DePaul's figures." The article followed with a chilling statement attributed to Ms. Shermer: "The way most procedures are performed today, most physicians make sure there's fetal demise."

Diana's figure came from Dr. Willard Cates, former chief of abortion surveillance for the Centers for Disease Control in Atlanta, as reported in the *Philadelphia Inquirer* on August 2, 1981. Cates estimated that 400 to 500 abortion live births occur every year in the United States.

Doubt surfaced again in various headlines: "Teen 'survived' abortion attempt" (the *Globe and Mail*, Toronto); "Gianna Jessen: 'Survivor's' Story" (*Yakima Herald-Republic*, Washington); " 'Saline survivor': Abortion is wrong" (*Gaston Observer*, North Carolina); "Abortion 'survivor' on tour delivering pro-life message" (*Rockford Register Star*, Illinois). A Minnesota newspaper, the *Star-Tribune*, not only implied that the fact of the abortion was suspect, but it also threw a shadow of suspicion on Gianna's character: "Girl calls herself an abortion survivor."

Gianna had told a reporter for the *Saint Cloud Visitor* (Minnesota), in an article published October 31, 1991, "People who are pro-choice are usually speechless when they hear my story." One pro-abortion person who was not speechless was Judy Maggio, a member of the executive board of the Rockford (Illinois) Coalition for Reproductive Choice. The article in the *Rockford Register Star* quoted her as saying that Gianna's appearance was an "appeal to the emotionalism of a second trimester abortion." (Gianna's birth weight, according to doctors, actually indicates she was aborted in the third trimester.)

Again, pro-abortionists challenged Gianna's story in the *Chicago Sun-Times* on December 12, 1991: "Nicki Nichols Gamble, a Planned Parenthood executive, questions whether Gianna's story is true. 'No doctor could legally perform a third trimester abortion unless the mother's life was at risk. The number of abortions performed at 24 weeks is minuscule. So even assuming the story is true, it's very non-representative. It tries to argue from the exception to the rule.' Planned Parenthood suspects that Gianna is being used as a 'poster child' counter-foil to Becky Bell. 'Becky isn't around to tell her story,' says Nichols Gamble."

Of course, neither are the vast majority of aborted children, whom Gianna represents. Nor are the other pregnant girls, like Becky, who have died from abortions—even legal ones—whether they were required to notify their parents or not. The real tragedy in Becky Bell's case is that abortion killed two people—not only the Bells' daughter, but also their grandchild, when *neither* death was necessary.

It's also strange that Ms. Nichols Gamble, an executive in Planned Parenthood, would not know that the 1973 Supreme Court ruling in Roe v. Wade legalized abortions for virtually *any* reason throughout all nine months of pregnancy, according to a Senate subcommittee in 1982. States are not allowed to forbid third-trimester abortions if the mother's health is at risk. And in Doe v. Bolton, decided the same day as Roe v. Wade, the Supreme Court defined *health* to include "all factors—physical, emotional, psychological, familial and the woman's age." If the Freedom of Choice Act ever passes, it would set unrestricted abortion throughout pregnancy in concrete.

When spokespersons for Planned Parenthood speak to the issue of Gianna's cerebral palsy, their words seem strangely paradoxical. Planned Parenthood of NW/NE Indiana issued a statement about Gianna that was quoted in the *Sunday Times* (Munster, Indiana) on March 1, 1992: "We have enormous compassion for this young woman. Certainly, her case is a tragedy in that she has suffered. However, this doesn't mean that every decision made to have an abortion is wrong.

"Women choose abortions for many reasons, sometimes out of despair. It is not possible to judge an entire issue based on this 14-year-old's experience. . . . Gianna is a symbol of triumph over adversity, not a symbol of why abortion should not be available."

The spokesperson did not explain how the organization could have tremendous compassion for the victim of a procedure they endorse, or how Gianna's suffering is a tragedy if the suffering of the victims who don't survive isn't. The spokesperson also didn't explain how the organization can see Gianna as a symbol of triumph over an adversity that they believe should remain a woman's right.

Attacks are also made on the motives behind Gianna's appearances. The *New York Times* said Gianna's story was "being shrewdly marketed . . . to keep passions high."

Jeffrey Zaslow devoted his column "All That Zazz" in the *Chicago Sun-Times* to Gianna on December 12, 1991. Under the title "Abortion survivor tells it from the kid's point of view," he dealt with the possibility that Gianna was being used. "Her mother," wrote Zaslow, "says Gianna won't allow anti-abortion groups to use her to raise funds. 'I watch carefully to make sure she's not exploited,' Diana says."

"If I had wanted to exploit Gianna," Diana told this author, "why didn't I haul her all around when she was a baby? Why did I wait till she was 12 to tell her she was aborted? Why did I let her decide whether to talk publicly about it? I've turned down invitations for her to appear on national talk shows, such as Phil Donahue, which I felt would sensationalize her story."

Gianna, too, is firm in wanting to tell her story but not engage in controversy. In the Zaslow interview, she said, "I don't want to debate. I won't have that. I'm just giving the message of love. . . . I'm not exactly trying to make them cry. But sometimes, they need a change of heart."

Despite her few detractors, response from her audiences is overwhelmingly positive. "People have come up and told me that they have had a change of heart," Gianna said in another interview. "They might have been for abortion before they came in the room, but they changed their mind when they left."

In an interview for the *Globe*, Gianna said, "Most of the people that come up to talk to me or shake my hand or hug me say they are so glad I survived. I'm very glad of that, too, but I think God saved me for His own reasons."

In another article, she said, "A lot of women tell me their whole life stories."

Teens respond, too. Gianna told a reporter for *The New American* (Dec. 31, 1991), "I talk about life as a teenager: the difficulties, challenges, peer pressure, the dangers of premarital sex. It's a message of hope—that whatever happens, even if it seems too difficult, don't give up, look to God for help. They come up to me and thank me. They send me letters. I find teenagers want to know the truth. I don't stand up here and preach to them, 'You can't do this, you can't do that.' I'm just talking to them as a friend, and they appreciate that."

Gianna doesn't seem too concerned about the controversy she stirs up everywhere. The author was sitting on the landing of Diana's house one day, where Diana has her desk and FAX machine, going through clippings while Diana was out shopping. Gianna came up the wrought iron stairs to the landing with two other teens in her wake. One was Jenny Morson, who met Gianna at the Youth Rescue in Atlanta and who was spending part of the summer with her. Jenny has freckles and long, dark hair with bangs. On a chain around her neck were two tiny, silver footprints—just the size of those made by a baby ten weeks into pregnancy.

The other girl was Jessi Oliver, Gianna's "all-time best friend" from junior high school in Valley Center. Jessi is tall and tan, with long, straight, honey-colored hair.

The girls reminisced about rescues. Gianna had been to several by then.

"Milwaukee was so scary," she said. "I was praying at this guy's feet—this pro-abort. He had, like, these steel boots, these huge Army boots, right next to my head. I prayed, 'Lord, please protect me!' My head was down, and his boot was right at my head. I was sure he was going to kick me. But he didn't."

She went on, "This police officer was stepping on Jenny's leg on purpose—like, really hard—and my other friend—don't write who it is—said 'Get off her leg!' He wouldn't, so she bit him!"

The girls laughed.

"I got lost every night," said Jenny.

Gianna explained, "She was driving because all her sisters were in jail for rescuing."

"How about at the L.A. rescue, when the clinic was in a building with all those other offices? The police thought this one man was the father of some kids that were rescuing, and they arrested him, too. He kept saying he was just there to take his wife to the podiatrist."

"Gianna," said Jessi, "remember when you patted that woman's stomach in Atlanta and she said, 'I'm not pregnant'?"

Gianna added, "That was the lady who went into the clinic and then changed her mind and didn't have an abortion after all. That was awesome!"

"Remember getting arrested in Atlanta?" Jessi asked.

"They threw Jenny in on top of us," Gianna said.

"They slid me into the car like a pizza into an oven," said Jenny, grinning.

"We're laughing now," Gianna said, "but when you rescue, it isn't a joke. We do it for Christ and for the babies."

The reporter looked back at the clipping from the *Los Angeles Times*. One paragraph stood out, a statement by Right to Life spokeswoman Nancy Myers: "Everyone gets tears in their eyes when Gianna stands there and says how glad she is to be alive. She's really an amazing person, very up—and it means something when this really cute, outgoing teenager says she's not a lump of tissue, that this is what abortion is all about—real people."

Precious people.

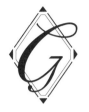

All Things Work Together

chapter 15

It was quiet in the San Clemente home on a January day in 1992. Gianna and her sister had flown to New York, where Gianna was scheduled to appear on NBC's "A Closer Look" with Faith Daniels. Robyn, the pregnant woman who lived with them, had given birth to a baby girl two days before and was still in the hospital. (Three months later, she moved out of Diana's house and got a place of her own.)

This time the author was there to interview Diana. She wanted to find out what makes Diana the kind of woman who values the very people society is insisting more and more loudly have no value. Why would a new single parent take into her heart and home a second daughter with cerebral palsy, a 96-year-old homeless man, an unmarried, pregnant woman with a small son, and three abused dogs?

Before she sat down, Diana found a large-print copy of *Reader's Digest* and placed it in Grandpa's hands. He was sitting at the table in the kitchen next to a large jukebox, the bright blue eyes in his wizened face peering at the women momentarily through the doorway.

"Here, Grandpa, I got you a book," Diana said.

He mumbled, "I don't know if I can . . ."

"It has large letters," Diana reassured him. "It has an article called 'Life on the Funny Farm.' It's just like our house." She laughed.

In a few minutes, the magazine slid off Grandpa's lap to the floor. He had fallen asleep.

"I had a wonderful, marvelous childhood," Diana began. She went on to describe how her parents, both Christian Scientists, had lived by the Golden Rule. Her dad, Harold Smith, was constantly helping people in need in her home-town of Anaheim, California. "I got lots of love and was close to both my parents, especially my father," she added.

When she was seven, her family adopted a 12-year-old boy. Four years later, the boy's two sisters moved in and stayed until they were 16. "Off and on, we had a lot of other people in and out of the house," Diana said. "We moved to a big house on a large piece of property on a dirt road—now a major highway—out in the rural part of Anaheim where Disneyland is today. Mom still lives there."

When she was 19, Diana's parents ended her idyllic youth by divorcing. "I had never even seen my parents argue, so it was traumatic," she said. "I rebelled. I rejected every-thing important to them, especially Christian Science.

"I moved in with five friends who were renting a big, plush apartment at the base of the Newport Pier. And even though I was engaged to a young soldier in Vietnam, I began dating another man—a divorced man with a five-year-old daughter! Jack was an investigator with the district attorney's office. He wouldn't come to the house because some of my friends did drugs. I eventually moved to my own little cottage in Laguna Beach"

When she turned 20, she quit work, bought a Mustang, and spent all her time at the beach. "I turned into a party animal," she said, shaking her head. "Every Friday night, we'd go drink and dance all night in Tijuana."

She eventually married Jack in Las Vegas. "Five months into our marriage, I got pregnant and had a miscarriage. I had to go to the hospital for a D and C. Because my family were Christian Scientists, I had never had an aspirin, had never been to a doctor except for the birth-control pills I was supposed to be taking. I thought sickness was always the result of doing something wrong."

The phone rang. It was Gianna, calling from New York. Apparently the interview at NBC hadn't gone well. Diana told her soothingly, "Trust me, when that gets out to the general public, it will turn around. I promise." Pause. "We'll just pray that God will use it, okay? Go have fun." Pause. "Don't worry about it. It will be fine. I love you, too."

When she hung up, she said, "There was a whole panel of pro-abortion people. She was almost the only pro-life person on it. She said they were really cold. But the people who watch will see through that."

After a pause, Diana returned to her own story. "In 1971, I got pregnant with Dené. Jack was doing undercover work all the time and also providing western White House security for President Nixon. Although we'd had problems, largely due to the all-consuming nature of his work, I thought our marriage was doing better. But one day we had a fight, and the next time I came home, Jack had moved out. The divorce sent me back into the party scene. I would pick Dené up at the baby-sitter, come home at night, feed her, and do all my motherly things. When she was asleep, I'd call in a teenage baby-sitter, and I'd go out and dance and drink, night after night."

When Dené was two and a half, Diana married Peter, who was 11 years her senior. It was the time of the Jesus Movement, and they lived in Laguna, where she saw a lot of street witnessing. "Laguna was full of weirdos, and to me, the 'Jesus freaks' were just part of it," Diana said.

"But a woman named Diane where I worked was always smiling," she continued. "I kept wondering why. I would watch her and think, *Maybe it's just because she drives a Mercedes.*" She laughed again.

Later, someone told her Diane was a Christian. Diana had always thought of herself as a Christian. But then a tragedy struck that made her willing to reconsider her beliefs. "One day, I got a call. My dad had suffered a heart attack and was in Tustin Hospital. He was comatose and was not expected to live.

"On Wednesday night, when I went to see him, my relatives were in his room arguing. I felt so stressed out and so alone that I walked out the front door of the hospital and across the street to a church. I could see lights on and hear voices inside. I stood in the courtyard and just stared at the name of the church, hardly aware of what I was doing.

"A woman came out and asked me, 'Are you all right?'

" 'Well, my dad's in a coma,' I said. 'He had a heart attack. He's not expected to live.'

" 'Would you like to speak to a pastor?'

" 'I'm going to be fine.' I was a Christian Scientist—I didn't see pastors!

"Gently, she persuaded me to come in, and I found myself sinking into a chair across from a man who started explaining the gospel. I didn't know what he was talking about. Where was Mary Baker Eddy?

"He talked a while and then asked, 'Would you like a personal relationship with Christ?'

"I said okay, and he prayed with me, but I was having a hard time concentrating. All I could think was, *Daddy's dying! Daddy, the man I run to whenever anything's wrong.*

"Before I left the church, the pastor warned me, 'Knowing Christ won't make your life easy.' I found that out when I got back to the hospital.

" 'Where were you?' my stepmother demanded. 'What if he'd died?' I didn't answer them aloud, but in my heart I said to God, 'I was across the street giving my life to You!'

"That night Daddy came out of the coma. I told him I loved him and that I forgave him for anything wrong he had done. He died two days later, but I remember having a kind of peace in spite of the pain.

"It was 1976. I was 29."

After that, she started going to church with Dené.

"I had been trying to adopt a little girl of mixed race who was developmentally disabled—one of Mom's foster kids,"

Diana went on. "But at the time, Peter and I were in the middle of moving, and we were turned down. I was crushed. But God put her into a perfect family, and my mother told me, 'God has a child perfect for you, too.'"

Some time later, Diana needed a total hysterectomy. The doctor told her afterward that medically speaking, she shouldn't have had even *one* child. That made her all the more thankful for Dené.

"On January 22, 1976, the anniversary of Roe v. Wade," Diana said, "at my church in Valley Center, I saw *The Silent Scream*, a film about abortion. I didn't know much about abortion. Some of my friends had had them; one ended up getting hepatitis. Not long after Roe v. Wade went into effect, another friend begged me to take her to the clinic. I did it to support her, not knowing what I was doing. I can remember sitting in the waiting room and seeing all those women who were going to have abortions and thinking, *Here I can't have any children, and these people are killing their children.*

"When I saw the film, I thought abortion was the most horrendous thing I had ever seen. The film motivated me to help the pro-life movement."

A few months later, she got a call from her mother. She had a new foster child in her home, a girl named Gianna.

"A Closer Look" aired three days later.

"It was scary," Gianna reported afterward, "sitting between people who thought abortion was okay. Faith Daniels was nice, but she seemed kind of callous. She wasn't mean, but it was like she had a wall up, you know, so she could do her business."

The show dealt with the abortion of viable fetuses— babies old enough to survive outside the womb. It featured five individuals in favor of late abortion—three men who make a living at it and two women who chose to undergo it because their unborn babies were severely handicapped. Seated between one of the abortionists and a woman who aborted her baby at five months, Gianna had reason to feel intimidated.

Besides Gianna, only two individuals on the panel, both male doctors, were against late abortion. Although Faith Daniels, who emcees the show, appeared impartial, those who defended abortion had twice as much air time as those who opposed it.

Gianna followed two of the doctors and the two mothers who had made agonizing decisions to abort. She was seated, smiling, wearing a red-and-blue-flowered print shirt. On the screen were her name and the words "Mother tried to abort her."

Instead of introducing Gianna as a survivor of a third-trimester abortion, Daniels introduced her as "an anti-abortion activist." Even though she asked Gianna to explain her "incredibly personal reason" for being against abortion, the understating of Gianna's unique perspective as a victim made her stand seem naive.

Gianna told her story, simply and earnestly. Then Daniels asked her opinion of the women who had spoken before her.

Gianna said she still thought abortion was wrong.

Later in the program, most of those who spoke from the audience lauded the women who had shown the "courage" to abort. One viewer expressed the opinion that not all handicapped children were as lucky as Gianna, that "being raised as a foster child" could be as bad as an abortion.

As Diana watched, she thought of her mother and the home she filled with love. *Should needing foster care be a capital offense?* she wondered.

After the program aired, Gianna found she had at least one supporter among the viewers. Cheryl in Florissant, Missouri, wrote her: "You did a great job, especially for a 14-year-old. I feel Faith Daniels really insulted you, . . . a person with a disability, when she asked if you thought it was okay for that other woman guest to abort her baby with a disability.

Me and my husband were so angry we couldn't see straight!"

Back home a few days later, Gianna curled up on the couch, describing to the author how terrible the show made her feel. "People think I come into contact with pro-aborts all the time, like it's no big deal for me, but I *don't.*"

She continued, "I have a tremendous fear of pro-abortion people 'cause I've seen them be so violent and so gross. I've had nightmares about this fear. I dreamed that I was lost in Paris, and these people were chasing after these rescuers. They spotted me in the crowd, and the pro-aborts took me and dragged me. They said, 'You're an abortion survivor, right?' and I said, 'Right,' and they were beating on me and all these terrible things. I deal with this day in and day out. I really do need prayer for this fear, because fear can stop so much."

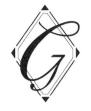

Reaching
Out
in Love

Gianna's rapport with those her own age makes her simple message of loving God, valuing life, and saving sex for marriage powerfully effective. For example, she drew 2,200 teens to a rally in Fremont, California.

Perhaps the most moving demonstration of Gianna's charisma, however, came the night she spoke to the congregation of the Christian Life Center in Yakima, Washington.

When she was introduced, she came on stage to the sound of bongo drums, singing "Everybody's got a seed to sow!" and interrupting herself to urge the audience, "You can clap louder than that! Keep it coming! Louder!"

Across the platform, down the stairs again, up one aisle and back, across the front of the church, stopping to stroke the face of a child in the front row, Gianna moved ceaselessly. "That's right, everybody! Come on!" she encouraged.

She went back on stage to sing "Fat Baby" and ended it breathless, saying abruptly, "I need water!" She explained to the audience, "I have a cold that I've been battling all day long, so you won't be surprised if I, like, faint. No, just joking! But I do have a cold, and I'm just trying my best and going to give this evening to the Lord."

A woman brought her water, and as she accepted it, Gianna told the audience, "Everybody in this lifetime goes through struggles, and it's hard, 'cause we feel like no one is there for us. Give your struggles to God and He will just fill you with love and joy and heal your wounds. In my young life, I have found this out, that if you don't give your hurts to the Lord, the wounds are going to get deeper and deeper until you are in a hole you feel you can never get out of.

"But God loves you, and there is no sin and no hurt that He cannot heal. That's why I'm going to sing 'Love Will Find You.' It says that no matter how lonely or broken you may be, no matter how dark you may feel inside, Jesus' love will reach out to find you." Then she sang the song.

She ended, winded. "God has brought me here to tell you a true story of how He worked in my life," she said. She gave her testimony, finishing up to applause, "Amen! Thank You, Lord! I really do feel I'm only here by the grace of God."

The audience applauded again; the people were really responsive.

"He's had a hand on my life from the beginning. He has a purpose for each of us. If the doctor had done his job right, I wouldn't be here. God turned something around that was meant for evil and turned it into good. And then He did an even greater miracle. He brought me to the place, as a child, where I understood that I was a sinner, but that He had loved me enough to provide a Savior—His Son, Jesus. When I trusted in Him to be my personal Savior and gave Him authority over my life, I not only found new strength and hope for here and now—I also got the promise that I'll spend forever with Him in heaven."

She spoke of her cerebral palsy. "In my foster home, I was just dead weight because of my disability, but I was a happy little girl. I still am. Sure I feel it when I hit the ground really hard or when I trip over my feet, especially in front of a cute guy. Otherwise, hey, I love it! I think God allowed it in my life to remind me that *He's* the one to be glorified. Not myself. So that's why I love it.

"I have been raised in a Christian home. That does not mean that my life has been a bowl of strawberries, but God has brought us through all the tough times. . . .

"I'm just a normal teenager. I eat too much junk food, I blast the Walkman in my ears. But I believe God has laid down a set of rules for us to live by, and I refuse to follow what everyone is telling all the teenagers today."

"Praise the Lord!" called out a man in the audience, and there was more applause.

Suddenly Gianna squinted up into the sound booth over their heads. "Mom?" she said. "Something just came to me. There are some kids in this audience, and I think the 'Baby' song would be good for them. What do you think?"

Apparently Diana approved, for Gianna started inviting the children to join her on stage. "I want all babies, toddlers— up to three or four—to come up here. Their parents can come, too. We're gonna put on our dancin' shoes!"

The little ones started coming, some with their mothers, others in twos and threes. She greeted each one with "Hi! How're you guys? Come on up," and she added, "You guys can stand around me. I don't want to fall over anybody."

The audience was starting to laugh. A baby in diapers was crawling up the steps. "Hi!" said Gianna. "Come on up!" The baby stopped, sat up, and began clapping. "Good," said Gianna with a grin. "You can just park it right there."

To each of those around her, she asked, "What's your name?"

Looking at her wide-eyed, they each breathed shyly into the microphone she was holding down to their mouths. Jessica, Lindsay, Mikey, Tia . . .

"Okay, kids, here we go. Hit the music, please! Let's dance!"

The music of Amy Grant's "Baby, Baby" began to play, and Gianna sang the lyrics, moving among the children and leaning down to sing to them, "I'm so glad you're mine!" The older ones sang with her. The younger ones stopped dancing as she approached to stare up at her, awed. One of the babies was swaying and clapping; Gianna kissed her on the cheek.

As the music faded, Gianna thanked them with delight. "Give 'em a hand!" she told the audience. The children filed back to their places—all but one. Gianna turned around, and there was a little girl still at her side.

"Hi! What's your name? Everyone, this is Tiffany!"

Once again she asked for water, and when it came, she drained the glass and gasped, "Thank you, Lord, for water!"

Her eyes sparkled. "We have to have audience participation, because if you don't participate, I'll come down *there* and make you come up *here!* I have a cordless microphone, and I can come down and see if you're not participating. This is a mellow song. I know I get a little rowdy at times, but hey"— with a coy sideways glance—"that's part of being a kid!

"I need you to do something kind of difficult because it's hot in here, but I need you to do it anyway. Put your arm around the person next to you. Everybody has to have an arm around someone. If you see someone without an arm around the person next to them, send them up to me.

"I heard a no! I have very sharp ears!" She limped down one aisle and addressed a little girl. "Want to come on up and put your arm around me? Okay! I've got a friend!" Not one but two little girls followed her back up on stage. Then two more, even littler.

"Any of the bigger ones?" asked Gianna. "I'm not strong enough to pick them up." There were children coming up the steps behind her. Then a teenage boy dragged his friend bodily to Gianna's feet. "I think I've made some friends forever!" she exclaimed.

Suddenly they were streaming from all over the auditorium, and the stage was soon full. Something very touching was happening. People weren't coming forward at an invitation to be saved. They weren't offering themselves for missionary service. They simply wanted to be near someone who loved them.

There was an acceptance here, a sense of "You can do it—but even if you can't, you still have value." Not a call to do. Just an affirmation that it was enough to be. Here was one who had been rejected and could still love, who had suffered and yet did not want revenge, who had been put to death and yet lived. A girl who limped and got colds and lost her train of thought and fell down at awkward moments—a girl as vulnerable as each girl there—and yet she thanked God for life.

"Anyone else? Feel free! This is cool! True audience participation! Any more teenagers out there wanta come hang with us?" They were still coming.

She began to sing "Friends." A row of girls toward the back swayed to the music. A smaller girl came up spontaneously and hugged Gianna's knees, almost throwing her off balance. Gianna stopped singing long enough to respond, "I don't want to fall down—I love you!"

By the time the song ended, Gianna had made her way back down to the foot of the platform. She turned to those above her and said, "Everyone here—up on stage or off stage—if you ever feel like you don't have any friends, you've got two—me and Jesus!"

She held the microphone close to her, as if it were something precious. "With this next song, I want everyone to feel God's love pouring out over them. I'd like it to become real for you."

It already had.

Among those to whom Gianna has reached out and who have reached out to her in turn are both the famous and the not-so-well-known. The former group includes Rush Limbaugh, Jack Hayford, Cal Thomas, and Oliver North. ("He's a wonderful man, so down to earth," Gianna reported.) Meeting such celebrities is one of the fringe benefits of her public appearances.

She said of her meeting with Michael W. Smith, one of her musical heroes, "I got to go to his house. He's really cute and really nice. His wife is real petite, and I met three of their kids. I sang 'Agnus Dei,' and he played for me. He told me, 'Gianna, keep your heart pure before God.'"

Naturally, Gianna has also met many leaders in the pro-
life movement. These include Randall Terry; Tim and
Beverly LaHaye; Pat Boone ("real laid-back," Gianna said);
Dr. and Mrs. Jack Willke, founders of Right to Life ("really
sweet people"); Joe Scheidler, founder of Pro-Life Action
League ("a dynamite guy"); Congressman Bob Dornan
("neat—really funny"); Father Paul Marx of Human Life
International ("hysterical"); and Carol Everett, a former
abortionist and author of *The Scarlet Lady* ("awesome—and
so much fun").

Shari Richard, an ultrasonographer who produced the
video *Ultrasound: A Window to the Womb* and who has testified before House and Senate subcommittees about life
within the womb, also makes high marks with Gianna. In
early September 1992, they were both speakers at "Life, the
Maine Event," a Right to Life banquet at which Diana was
honored with a plaque as their mother of the year.

"Ultrasound has disproved the 'blob of tissue' theory,"
Shari told the audience. "Our technology just wasn't sophisti-
cated enough to see those teeny fingers and toes before.

"In October 1989, at a National Abortion Rights Action
League workshop, 'Framing and Selling the Pro-Choice
Message,' Harrison Hickman said, 'Probably nothing has
been as damaging to our cause as technological advances that
show pictures of the fetus.' "

Gianna said of Shari, "She's real sweet, real tender-
hearted for God, one of those people who show you that even
if you have struggles in life, don't give up."

In mid-September, Gianna appeared with the syndicated
columnist Cal Thomas at a Crusade for Life rally in Santa
Barbara, California. Afterward, Thomas wrote about her in
his column: "Pro-choice activists and their soulmates in
Congress and in the press are treating the likelihood of Judge
Clarence Thomas' confirmation to the Supreme Court as
they might a visit from Freddie Krueger, the main character
in the *Nightmare on Elm Street* movies," he said.

"Columnists Ellen Goodman, Richard Cohen and Anna Quindlen—part of the 'don't mess with my body' brigade—are sounding apocalyptic warnings, raising the specter of coat hangers and bleeding women in back alleys. . . .

"Quindlen and the other hysterical commentators . . . should meet 14-year-old Gianna Jessen. . . .

"Anna Quindlen says it is insulting to tell a woman she can't abort her unborn child. A greater insult is to tell someone like Gianna Jessen she is a mistake, the result of a botched abortion who ought to be dead. . . .

"Why was Gianna Jessen not considered a person while inside her mother but seconds later, as she emerged gasping for breath, she inherited the full protection of the law? This is the stuff of which nightmares are made."

After meeting him, Gianna described Thomas as "very nice. He has an extremely dry sense of humor. I didn't know when to take him seriously, so I laughed at everything he said."

Just as much fun as meeting celebrities, though, is making friends around the world and receiving their letters. The letters are from kids in high school, junior high, and elementary school. Many of them say they are home schooled, as Gianna is. They saw her on TV or read about her in a magazine.

They're shy; they're bold. They call her Gianna and Gina and Jana and Lady Gianna and Ms. Jessen and Miss Jensen. They tell her about their families. ("I have a brother and a sister, and both of them are pains!" wrote Rochelle, ten, from Williamsport, Pennsylvania.) They write about their pets, their favorite colors, their favorite singers. They draw pictures for her or enclose school photos. They tell her their ambitions. Many of them express deep concerns and ask Gianna's advice on intimate problems.

From Theresa, 11, of Rochester, New York: "I have an 8 people family. Starr + Rebecca are adopted. Both were going to be aborted. I am almost 12 years old but have been involved in the pro-life movement since before I could walk.

My mom hung pro-life signs on my stroller."

From Shannon, 16, of Newark, California: "When you were saying how hard it can be to be a teenager in this world and that sometimes it really can feel like no one understands what you're going through and no one cares—it was exactly how I felt. It was as if you were speaking directly to me. God is awesome. I love it when He does that! Thank you for sharing that with *me* and many others who were hurting."

From Julie, 16, of Roanoke, Virginia: "I went to the CPC banquet here in Roanoke. My dad told me that Oliver North and a woman who had been aborted and survived were both going to speak. . . . I pictured an old lady with curly white hair in a wheelchair. What a pleasant surprise to find out it was a girl my own age! Everyone in Roanoke was buzzing about how totally cool you are. *You stole the show!*"

From Donald, 25, a man with cerebral palsy in Goleta, California: "My case is a little more severe than yours—I get around on crutches, and I can't nearly sing like you can!—but I can identify with you in that by God's hand and His grace I am living an active life, even though sometimes I feel so incapacitated and limited.

"I was surprised to learn there are people who have survived being aborted, and this knowledge has reinforced my convictions about abortion. I'm glad that you are out there as a living demonstration of the preciousness of life."

From a teenager in Canton, Michigan, on behalf of her little sister: "Our names are Sandra and Danae. I am 14 and she is 6. We saw the article about you in *Brio* magazine. It said that when you were 10, you had surgery. We think, judging from the way you described it, that Danae will be having the same operation . . . a rhizotomy. Danae's been very nervous about it, and we thought it would help to talk to someone who's had the surgery. We would appreciate it if you would write back to us."

After Danae's surgery, Gianna met her and her sister in Detroit. Diana told a reporter, "The relationship between the two sisters reminds me so much of Dené and Gianna—the older sister watched over the younger so lovingly."

Phil, 31, of Bellefonte, Pennsylvania, wrote from prison: "I needed to tell you how you brought a bright ray of sunshine in my heart!! I am sitting in a PA State Prison at the moment. . . .

"One morning, I was changing channels on my T.V., when I was captured by your innocence and your smile. Every time you smiled, I felt a healing salve flow through my spirit. (You made me cry!)

"I was adopted by a family also, Gianna—when I was 2. Yet I was still not wanted. I don't know what a loving family is, but I have felt touches of Love.

"You went inside me and took away the pain."

From Brandi, 15, of Maryland: "I'm sure you don't remember me. I met you when you talked at Loyola and the youth rally. You signed my jeans. I had to write to tell you what a great person you are. You really helped me see that I didn't need to search for my biological father!"

Jim, 17, of Hazelton, North Dakota, enters speech competitions with a talk about abortion. He ends his speech by discussing Gianna. He wrote her: "They cry when I talk about the procedures and when I tell them . . . your story. I would like to have a photo of you to [blow] up. It would serve as one of my illustrations and do more than any graph or chart ever would."

And a note from Jamie, 15, of Fremont, California, provided comic relief: "So how long have you been in show biz?"

Gianna even received a marriage proposal from a man in India.

"I wish I could answer all the letters I get," sighs Gianna. "I read every one I get, and I want people to know that. But it's hard for me to *write* letters. Some of them are really deep and emotional, too, and they want advice. *I* don't know what they should do! But praying is always a good start."

Diana answers as many of the letters as she can, particularly those that ask questions or seem urgent. Gianna, once again the typical teenager, loves to respond by phone to teens she has befriended at her concerts.

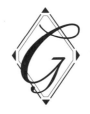

Unexpected
Clues

chapter 17

It was the middle of August 1992—and the middle of a heat wave that had been scorching Southern California for a week, with temperatures over 100 degrees. Diana had spent the morning shopping and managed to find two large suitcases for Gianna and herself. As she came out of the store, the smell of plump, meaty hot dogs cooking filled the air. Diana realized she was ravenous. Why go home for lunch?

Hauling the suitcases with her, she stepped into the short line of people waiting for food under the red-white-and-blue-striped umbrella in front of the store. The woman ahead of her glanced back and smiled.

"You must travel a lot," she said.

"I do—for the pro-life movement." Diana watched the woman's face and thought she saw her start. *That will probably kill that conversation,* she thought with a sigh.

The woman seemed to read her mind. "It's okay," she said. "I'm Catholic. What exactly do you do?"

"Well, I have a real different story. I adopted my daughter after she had been aborted."

Diana wasn't imagining it this time. The woman started, then turned to face her and demanded with interest, "Is your mother Penny?"

"Yes! How did you—"

"And your daughter is Gianna?"

"Yes!"

"I knew her and her birth mother!"

"You're kidding!"

The woman was eager to talk. "Before the birth mother

lost custody of her—do you remember that case back in 1978, when Dr. William Waddill from Westminster was accused of smothering a baby who survived one of his abortions?"

"Yes," said Diana. "The trial was in all the papers. Someone sent me the clippings. They're somewhere in my garage."

"Did you know," asked the woman, "that Gianna was at that trial?"

Now it was Diana's turn to look startled. "No!"

"Gianna was just a year old. Her birth mother and I smuggled her up the back stairs of the courthouse and into the trial. The birth mother testified in court that there was an expert witness present who had survived abortion."

Diana dug the file out of the garage when she got home. The details of the abortion sounded uncannily like Gianna's. Dr. Waddill had performed a saline abortion on a teenager seven months pregnant, and the baby girl was born alive.

But then, according to the testimony of a nurse, the doctor interrupted her efforts to help the baby's breathing. A fellow physician testified that he saw Waddill choke the infant. "I saw him put his hand down on this baby's neck and push down," said Dr. Ronald Cornelson. "He said, 'I can't find the trachea,' and 'This baby won't stop breathing.' " The baby was dead by the time she reached the hospital.

"Surviving 'Fetus' Stirs Dispute" ran the headline of an article in the *National Catholic Register* dated April 23, 1978. It began, "A one-year-old baby girl who survived a saline abortion attempt was brought to the witness stand April 5 by her mother, who was called by the prosecution to testify in the two-month-old murder trial of Dr. William B. Waddill, Jr.

"The 18-year-old mother was identified as 'Miss Hobbs' and the child as 'Margo Hobbs' by prosecuting attorney Robert Chatterton."

Margo Hobbs was Gianna! Diana realized. Gianna had been aborted by a different doctor only a month before Dr.

Waddill aborted the baby who subsequently died. Diana read on. Apparently Dr. Waddill testified that the baby he aborted, if it had survived, would have been "totally brain damaged." So Gianna was the prosecution's "exhibit A" to prove that survivors of saline abortion could be relatively normal and healthy.

Waddill's attorney, also a physician, called this a "cheap shot." "That baby is not normal," he said, indicating Gianna. "She has cerebral palsy."

After two mistrials, the *Register* ran an article titled "Waddill: Is He Off the Hook?" In it, the one holdout at the second trial confided that his eleven peers, who voted for acquittal, had made comments that the baby was "as good as dead" anyway because her mother wanted her dead through the abortion.

Charges against Waddill were dismissed.

Diana held a clipping in each hand and gazed into space. *That could have been Gianna*, she thought. *That baby girl was aborted alive and didn't quite make it to the hospital. But Gianna did.* She was struck anew with the conviction that God had intervened and spared Gianna for a purpose.

Who had rushed Gianna from the clinic to the hospital? Who had saved her life? In spite of all the publicity surrounding Gianna, no one had ever stepped forward to fill in that piece of the puzzle.

Gianna believed it was an angel.

The front door to Diana's home was wide open. Intensely indigo morning glories lined the front walk and covered the garage wall. The reporter followed six-inch hoses and cords from a noisy truck parked in the street up to the door and knocked.

Diana was talking on a portable phone. Her face lit up when she saw the reporter, now a friend, and she motioned her in. There was furniture piled in the tile entryway.

As Diana put the phone down, she indicated a man who

was vacuuming the living room and explained, "We're having the carpets cleaned. The dogs are out back. Grandpa is at day care."

"Day care?"

"Three days a week. I felt kind of scared wheeling him up the ramp onto the bus, but he seems to like it."

Gianna greeted the reporter from the circular wrought-iron steps. "I remember getting on the bus that way. On the whole bus, there was only one seat for a person not in a wheelchair. The day I was able to sit in that seat was great!"

"Gianna wrote a song for Grandpa," Diana said.

Gianna sang it softly:

> I saw a brother of mine on the street today,
> For what reason, it's hard to say.
> I stood and watched as he begged for change,
> But people walked on by not even caring
> if he lived or died.
> Old man, I've got some bread for you.
> Old man, hang on, I'll get some water, too.
> Believe in Him and you'll never go hungry again.
>
> © Gianna Jessen
> Used by permission.

Gianna writes many of her own lyrics and sings them to friends, who translate the sounds into notes. Sometimes it irks Gianna that reporters and talk-show hosts focus so much on the fact she was aborted. "They overlook my music, and that's sometimes irritating. There's more to me than the story of how I came into the world. I'm a musician."

One newspaper account put the emphasis where Gianna wants it: "Abortion may be her crusade, but music is her passion."

"The idea for 'Written in the Sky' just popped out of the sky one day," according to Gianna, while she and her mother were driving home from a testimonial appearance. "I chose the title because I believe every lyric was given to me from God—almost as if I look up and *pow!*—there are all the words right before me."

"Little Toys," a song Gianna and Diana co-wrote in 1992, "is a real sappy song," Gianna told the *Philadelphia Inquirer* candidly, "but it's a real convincing song."

Now she addressed the amiable, curly-haired man in the living room. "You've cleaned our carpets before, haven't you?"

He switched off his machine to hear her. "Once," he answered with a smile.

"You do a rad job!"

"Thank you."

"Isn't this a crazy household?"

His smile broadened, but he said only, "A little bit."

Diana looked across the room at him, her arms akimbo. "I could never get married again," she told the reporter. "Where could I find a husband who would put up with all this?"

From the steps, Gianna told the latest that God had done for her. "Last night, I was crying because I couldn't figure out how to multiply fractions, and I have a math placement test today. I get so frustrated when I can't learn something. I have a friend going into pre-algebra, and I can barely do the basic things. I prayed that God would help me understand. And this morning I just opened the book and looked at it, and I understood it! Praise the Lord!"

So how is "airplane school"?

"Well, I missed eighth-grade graduation of all the home-schoolers—I was supposed to sing there—because the plane was late leaving San Francisco. It broke down three times before it took off."

"I had just bought her the cutest graduation dress in Atlanta," added Diana.

"I wore it the next day to Jessi's graduation instead."

Diana is hardly a strict schoolmarm, but she does try to fit

Gianna's education into the cracks. Before visiting a new place, Diana has its Chamber of Commerce send information. In Spain, they toured a cathedral, and she had Gianna write a report about its history when they came home. They stopped at a plantation in Louisiana to let Gianna pick cotton.

"I couldn't believe I was standing there picking cotton!" Gianna confided afterward. "But it's good to see things that you read about in your textbooks. And I've learned how to get along with all kinds of people. It's just a good growing experience. But sometimes I just wish I could go to high school, meet a guy, and be able to be near him every day."

Gianna and Dené would be leaving for Virginia the next morning. Gianna went upstairs to pack, calling down over the noise of the shampooer, "Can I take my overalls—the silky ones?"

"No, no, no!" Diana called back. "You're going to be with Oliver North!"

Gianna had not yet met North at that time. Nonetheless she replied, "I get to be with Oliver North? That's great!"

Meanwhile, Diana told the reporter about the "divine serendipity" in meeting the woman who had helped smuggle Gianna into the Waddill trial. The reporter took the clippings about the trial up to Gianna's small room off the landing with its posters—seven of Amy Grant, two of Michael W. Smith—on the walls and on the sloped ceiling.

The reporter sat in the wicker chair and read about the trial while Gianna, who had finished packing, sat at her desk, studying predicate nouns for the English placement test she had to take before the flight. She started to turn a page and thought of something. "Who is Oliver North?" she asked.

Like Diana, the reporter held the clippings and stared into space. The horror of what could have happened faded and was replaced by the sounds of Lobo barking, the telephone and FAX lines ringing, and Gianna reviewing grammatical rules. She remembered how Gianna laughingly described herself once: "I'm just an ordinary kid who came into the world in an extraordinary way," pointing out that God could bring good out of it.

The reporter borrowed the worn Bible on Gianna's desk to look up the verse to which she had alluded: Genesis 50:20. "You intended to harm me," Joseph told the brothers who sold him into slavery, "but God intended it for good to accomplish what is now being done, the saving of many lives."

In the next room, Diana was about to administer the placement tests. Gianna was asking, "Can we pray?" and Diana petitioned the Lord conversationally to give Gianna wisdom and peace.

Perhaps because of Gianna, the reporter thought, *God will save many lives.*

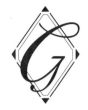

A
Gathering
of Survivors

Wherever she went, Gianna was always eager to know, "Are there any more like me?" The answer is yes.

Heidi Huffman, a year younger than Gianna, survived a suction abortion. She wrote from Spartanburg, South Carolina, signing herself "F.A.S.—Fellow Abortion Survivor." Monty Bowman of Winona Lake, Indiana, and Sarah Smith, who was interviewed with Gianna on a cable show in Oregon, had each survived the abortion of a twin. Gianna heard of others who had been severely impaired, physically or mentally, by abortion procedures. Ana Rosa Rodriguez, for example, had an arm pulled off in utero by a doctor attempting to abort her.

When Vern Kirby of Human Life International (HLI) heard about Gianna in 1991, he, too, wondered if there were any other abortion survivors. So he advertised and found survivors all around the world and invited them to come together, for the first time in history, to discuss what had happened to them.

The First International Gathering of Abortion Holocaust Survivors was held as an adjunct to the Eleventh World Conference on Love, Life and Family on April 29—May 3, 1992. It was sponsored by HLI in Ottawa, Canada. Scholars, priests, nuns, dignitaries, and lay people attended from 58 countries. Security was tight because vocal, organized opposition to the conference made violence a real possibility.

The conference opened on Wednesday night with Mass at Saint Patrick's. As the service ended, Knights of Columbus

171

in black and crimson capes and plumed caps, swords drawn, led the way out of the church. Then came Father Paul Marx, 71, founder and president of HLI, described by a local newspaper as "portly, cherubic . . . resembling nothing so much as an aging biker on vacation." Behind him were 1,500 pro-lifers carrying candles.

TV floodlights blinded the marchers, and their hymns and prayers were drowned out by the jeers, insults, and sing-song slogans of 500 pro-abortionists. They held signs reading "Shock the Right," "Queers for Choice," "Pagans for Choice," "Keep your rosaries off our ovaries," and "Racist, Sexist, Anti-Gay, Born-Again Bigots Go Away" in both English and French—and pictures of a naked woman hanging Christlike on a coat hanger.

Fifty Ottawa police on foot, in cars, on motorcycles, and on horseback interposed themselves between the two groups. All the way up Kent Street to Wellington Street, then up to the Parliament building on a hill overlooking the city, they marched without incident.

A letter from a man named Robert Lyman to the *Ottawa Citizen* afterward noted, "Anyone who saw the demonstration knows there was a remarkable contrast between the behavior of the groups. The pro-life group walked, prayed and sang hymns in a way that deliberately avoided provocation. The 'pro-choice' group was raucous, loud, abusive and hostile."

Early Friday morning, eight abortion survivors, seated at a long table in the penthouse of the Skyline Hotel, met with journalists. Behind them hung flags of the world, and above, a large, red sign reading "Abortion Holocaust Survivors." Later in the day, they would participate in a panel discussion, and there would be a banquet in their honor the following night.

Vern Kirby explained to the media the purpose for the survivors' presence: "They have a very powerful message, a very moving message. The other side tries to de-personalize the debate by labeling fetuses as non-human. What this does is re-personalize it . . . by having human beings here today."

The youngest survivor was 17-month-old Lauren Pulliam—blonde, blue-eyed, in a frilly red-plaid dress, with white teddy bear and bottle nearby. The oldest was Ladislav Mlejnek, a 65-year-old man from Eastern Europe who spoke Esperanto. Each one had a miracle to relate.

Those who were old enough told their own stories, some through translators. Lauren's grandmother spoke for her.

"As a Birthright volunteer," she said, "I had run pregnancy tests on many young women. But on a Sunday night in April, when I ran one for our 17-year-old daughter, it felt like my heart was in my mouth, and my hands trembled. The test was positive. She and I looked at each other in disbelief, and she began to cry."

Urged by counselors at Planned Parenthood to do so, Lauren's young mother chose abortion. Four weeks later, a nurse told her she was still pregnant. Despite the Planned Parenthood staff's attempt to schedule her for a resuction, she went to a gynecologist, who let her hear her daughter's heartbeat and watch her motions via ultrasound. Lauren was born full-term and normal.

Mlejnek's father, an atheist, persuaded his wife to have a German doctor perform an abortion on her in 1927. When she found out she was still pregnant, the doctor discovered she had been carrying twins.

A Colombian lady, Hilda Espitia, survived her mother's attempts to abort her in 1945 using herbal concoctions.

In her seventh month of pregnancy, Marilyn Miller's mother used chemicals and then an injection from a doctor to abort her. Marilyn, who had appeared with Gianna on "The Maury Povich Show," was delivered alive in a bedpan.

Linda Noie spoke on behalf of her 13-year-old son. Linda was a recently divorced mother of two when she became pregnant in 1979. She went to an abortion clinic at her boyfriend's insistence and underwent an abortion, praying that, somehow, the Jesus she didn't really know would work a miracle. She had to return to the clinic twice because of complications, but the symptoms only worsened, and the clinic staff decided she must have a tumor. When Linda consulted another doctor, she, too, found out she was still pregnant. She gave birth to Joshua five months later and found Jesus through pro-lifers.

Patricia Case, a 43-year-old from California, told how she had felt rejected all her life and had never understood why until, in response to her suicide attempt, her mother confided that she had tried to abort Pat three times.

When it was her turn to tell her story, Gianna said, "I came here along with the other survivors to show that there is life in the womb and no one has a right to take it away. People are saying we were just blobs of tissue."

Later, she expanded that thought: "I went through [abortion], and I survived it. I wasn't a blob of tissue, I wasn't a sprout or anything, I was a baby. . . . I believe that people need to know the truth. There's a lie going around that babies in the womb are a blob of tissue. God doesn't make us kind of burst into a human being when we come out."

Denise Lachance, spokeswoman for Pro-Choice Network, objected in the *Citizen*, "[HLI] is really a political movement dressed in religious clothing. It's all right for them not to have abortions. But they don't have the right to impose their ideas on others."

In the *Ottawa Sun*, Lachance "dismissed the 'survivor' gathering as a 'cheap media stunt.'

"We know who the real abortion holocaust victims are—the women who died from back street abortions, from self-induced abortions in their bathrooms. What this really shows is the crying need for access to legal abortion early in pregnancy."

Reporters challenged the survivors with these accusations. Pat Case rejected the suggestion by reporters that the meeting was just a publicity stunt. "I don't feel like a star," she said. "We're just here to say what happened to us. We exist. That's the reality."

One male reporter asked Gianna if she thought she was

being exploited by anti-abortionists. A local paper reported her answer as "I'm not an adult, but I'm old enough to know that abortion is murder."

The *Globe and Mail* made it more dramatic: "14-year-old Gianna Jessen's eyes flash with anger at the suggestion she is being manipulated by anti-abortion groups when she talks publicly about how she survived an abortion. 'I may not be an adult, but I have a right to say what I think,' snapped Gianna."

"I talked back to that reporter," Gianna confided to a friend afterward, " 'cause he was sarcastic. I said, 'If I'm old enough to have an abortion, I'm old enough to speak out against it.' Everyone applauded. Afterward he said to me, 'No need to get all hot around the collar.' "

In private, Diana felt parents bringing younger children did verge on exploitation: "I feel they shouldn't have their children speak until they're older and can make their own decision."

Dr. Margaret Somerville, director of McGill University's Centre for Medicine, Ethics and Law, although concerned about the effect on survivors of being brought to the conference by parents, told the *Citizen* the gathering was an "immensely effective" psychological approach to the abortion debate: "When you recognize that you would have killed this person, who is now standing before you, you're quite horrified by the thought that that's what you would have done. It's a very powerful message."

The question of exploitation had come up before. In Minnesota, Marna Johnson, executive director of the Abortion Rights Council, had said, "I can certainly understand why this young woman is personally opposed to abortions. But to parade her around and to try to personify her as the thing that is wrong with abortion is terribly exploitive."

Nancy Koster of Minnesota Citizens Concerned for Life had countered, "The person that exploited her was the person that tried to kill her."

In North Carolina, a few days after the HLI conference,

it would come up again. The *Gaston Observer* recorded,
"[Gianna] wants to share her story with others. 'She's doing
what she feels God called her to do,' said her mother. 'I don't
coach her. I feel she has the right to speak or not to speak,
because she knows her emotional strength.' "

The article went on, "Gianna says, 'I've been called a
freak-show, a pro-life cheerleader and they say my mom's a
pro-life activist with a prop.' . . .

"But she doesn't listen to critics, she said, because there
are so many people who come up to her, some with tears in
their eyes, and thank her for speaking out.

" 'I'm just telling a story of God's love,' she said. 'I'm not
there to condemn.' "

The name-calling Gianna referred to didn't seem to
bother her. In *USA Today* on January 22, 1992, Kate
Michelman, head of the National Abortion Rights Action
League, accused anti-abortionists of "parading Gianna
around like she's some kind of sideshow freak for the cause."
Mark Davis, a talk-show host on WRC Radio in
Washington, D.C., was the one who called Diana "a pro-life
activist with a prop."

Newsweek referred to Gianna as a "pro-life cheerleader"
in an April 27 article titled "Abortion's Long Siege": "There
is even a traveling ministry dedicated to publicizing the
unique situation of Gianna Jessen of San Clemente, Calif., a
15-year-old girl whose mother tried to abort her; she survived
but suffered mild cerebral palsy. Now, with her adoptive
mother Diana DePaul, she travels the country as a pro-life
cheerleader and speechmaker, spreading a message of 'education and forgiveness.' "

As "A Closer Look" had, *Newsweek* chose the odd phrase
"tried to abort her." The *Ottawa Sun* on April 29 called the
abortion "unsuccessful." Both phrases imply that abortion
involves not just termination of a *pregnancy*, but also termination of the life of the *baby*—that an abortion is not complete
unless a fetus is not just removed, but also destroyed.

Gianna has commented in interviews that "if the doctor had done his job right, I wouldn't be here." Perhaps someone needs to clarify exactly what it is a pregnant woman has a right to when she pays for an abortion: a terminated pregnancy or a dead baby.

Comparing herself to the others she met, Gianna said after the conference, "I thought I was real different—I had a different perspective from the other survivors or mothers at the conference. God has given me joy in this ministry. Some of those from other countries were totally joyous, but those from our country were upset about their situation—even though they didn't have disabilities. I think it's important to be happy that we are here and not dwell on the fact we almost died."

Father Paul Marx summed up the importance of the Gathering of Abortion Holocaust Survivors: "Perhaps modern historians should apologize to Hitler for vilifying him as the worst demon the twentieth century has produced. The fact is, in terms of numbers of victims, cultural damage, and the sheer inhumanity of their methods and motives, the pro-abortionists of our current day take precedence."

Hitler labeled Jews and others "inferior" or "nonhuman" as an excuse to exterminate them, Marx pointed out. "Abortionists do the same thing with unborn children. Our gathering in Ottawa showed those certainly are human beings; they are not 'blobs of tissue' as abortionists claim. They were small human beings who now are bigger human beings.

"It was, after all, the testimony of survivors . . . coupled with photographs from the death camps, that helped shock the world into realizing the horrors of the Nazi Holocaust."

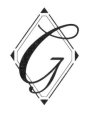

Looking for Gianna's Birth Mother

P at Rutherford, the investigator recruited by Rich Buhler to try to find Gianna's birth mother, is a Santa Claus look-alike. When he reunites people with lost relatives, biological parents, and childhood sweethearts, many people are convinced he *is* Santa Claus. He loves the role.

Facing the reporter as she pushed open the door of WorldWide Tracers was a bulletin board as big as the wall to which it was attached, covered with a collage of snapshots—people in groups of two or more, all happy. Pat Rutherford, a large, amiable man with a neatly trimmed gray beard, shook her hand and explained Reunion Wall.

"These are some of the 10,000 people we have brought together so far," he said. "We have lots of happy endings. This year we'll do 400-500 reunions—that's a little over one a day.

"It's really finding missing heirs that keeps us in business. We charge 30 to 50 percent of the inheritance. We had a couple who fled from Russia to Iran, France, and Brazil before they finally settled in the United States. They loved each other, but they had no children.

"Then the husband got Alzheimer's, and one day when his wife asked him to put shoes on, he choked her to death. He died shortly afterward of a broken heart, and their estate was left to two of the wife's sisters back in Russia. It was my job to find the sisters.

"I started in the Russian community in Los Angeles. Several people knew the couple and told me the story in tears. I got information about the sisters there, but I couldn't reach them through the Soviet government.

"Finally, I wrote a nasty letter to the Russian embassy, accusing their bureaucrats of being worse than ours. That did it! They cleared the way for me to get in touch with the sisters and give them their inheritance.

"We've made as much as $90,000 from a missing heirs case. But I'm not interested in making huge amounts of money. I've had fancy cars, my own plane, a large home, and it never brought me happiness. The company isn't designed to bring in a lot of money, but we sure bring happiness. We found two young children who were heirs to a $50,000 trust from their great-grandmother. They were the son and daughter of a migrant cantaloupe picker up north, living in utter poverty. They were able to buy a house with it. I still hear from their mother."

He gestured around him at shelves and shelves of volumes. "I've got every phone book in the country. If you were ever married or divorced in California, you're in my records. If you went to college, I've got the institution on microfiche. I've got census records, court records, military records, *Who's Who*. I've got your license plate number. I've got your old phone numbers.

"I don't care where you are. If I've got your name and date of birth, no matter where you are in the world, I've gotcha!" He grinned. "One time, all we had to go on was a lovesick guy's description of a 'girl in a blue dress' he had met in a barroom in Las Vegas. We found her.

"We have to be part detective, part 'I Spy,' and part CIA. We've found people the police couldn't find. We found two girls missing for 17 years—in 29 days. One woman had been looking for her natural mother for five years. I used voter records and found her in 20 minutes. Our most difficult case took eight months. We have a 98 percent success rate, and no case is ever closed—ever—until we find the person, dead or alive.

"I do a lot of young people who were on drugs. Runaways.

The mother or father will call, and the first thing they say is, 'I know he's dead.' And 99 percent of the time, he's not dead. A lot of times, the kid's just ashamed to go home. One man disappeared when he was 22, and we were put on the case 15 years later. His parents missed him, and he couldn't understand why, because he had stolen money from them. He was sure they'd never want to see him again.

"We had a man who left his wife and kids, went all the way across the country, remarried, had more kids, started a whole new life. When we found him, he thought his parents or ex-wife were after him. I told him no, everyone was just worried about him. He started crying and said, 'I really didn't think anybody cared.'

"I only do adoptions because God says do 'em. They're not profitable for us—we usually charge $650—and they can be gut-wrenching. You really get involved. People with nobody sometimes find they have a whole family. I think it's a misconception that birth parents don't want to meet the children they've put up for adoption. Of 4,000 cases, I've only had a few say no.

"I won't take a case unless I make the final connection myself. If parents are scared, I encourage them to take their time, to call me when they're ready. I've had movie stars ask me to find children they had out of wedlock. I've had women who were only 13 when they had a baby and had to give it up for adoption. The hardest ones to find are babies who were sold on the black market, because there's no record."

His office had just enough room for a desk, a bulletin board of his personal finds, and a large, glass case filling one wall. Rutherford waved the reporter to the one guest chair and took a seat behind his desk, leaning back with his arms behind his head.

"I was never a gun collector," he said, "but people would come to me and ask me to find somebody for them, and they'd say, 'I don't have any money, but I do have this old gun.' That one over there in the case is a rifle that went up

San Juan Hill with Teddy Roosevelt. There's a genuine Bowie knife in there, too, from the Alamo. Somebody traded it to me for finding a relative.

"The gun behind you, above the door, is a Kentucky muzzle loader from the days of Davy Crockett. They'd stomp the powder and ball down the barrel with a big, wooden rod, and then the rod becomes part of the gun. I've got ten or 15 of 'em now—you know Texans. What'll I do with 'em in heaven? Maybe the Lord'll let me shoot 'em on the Fourth of July."

"Texas?"

"Raised in San Antonio, worked in Dallas. A patriot—loved my country and made bombs for the defense department. Then I became a Christian, and I thought, 'Gee, them bombs hurt people! I want to make people happy.'

"Someone sent me a book about a man who tracked down people who had government money coming to them. I read it and thought, *That sounds like fun.* So I moved to California and started WorldWide Tracers.

"When I met Rich Buhler, I was just one man in a little office doing my own thing. He's had me on his show 'Table Talk' about ten times and has referred people like Diana to me, and now I have staffs in 12 offices: Salem, Arkansas; Kankakee, Illinois; Hyannis, Massachusetts; Tulsa, Oklahoma; Portland, Oregon; two in Texas; five in California.

"I'm 65, and I should be retiring, but I love my work. I'm so thankful I have a ministry where we put people together. We cry. We laugh—"

He stopped. "So," he said, "you want to know about Gianna's mom." He leaned forward, said "Excuse me," and bellowed over the reporter's head, "Jeanie?" When a woman appeared at the door, he said, "Bring me the file on Gianna Jessen."

While she was gone, the reporter asked, "Have you found the biological mother?"

"We're that close to finding her. We know her name and her last place of residence and the place she works."

Jeanie came back with a thin manila folder.

"Thanks." He took it from her and opened it, glancing over the few pages it contained. "I'll tell you right now that the facts of the birth don't support the story."

"What do you mean?" the reporter asked.

"I mean, I got copies of the hospital records, and it doesn't look to me like there was any abortion. Someone has penciled in 'premature birth' over the word *abortion*."

"Couldn't that have been added to protect the abortionist?"

"Sure it could." He leaned forward, elbows on the desk, fingers laced. "But you want to know what I think? Doesn't Gianna's mother take her all over and have her speak for groups and things? I think it makes a good story. I'm not trying to say she's just trying to make money off of her—but, you know, it sounds good, and it helps the pro-life cause—"

"I've come to know Diana pretty well," the reporter interrupted, "and I don't think she's the kind of woman who would deliberately deceive."

"I've met her, too," Rutherford said. "She's a real nice lady. I'm not saying it's deliberate, necessarily—maybe that's what she was told and she really believes it. I'm just saying that's not what the records seem to indicate."

Rutherford had turned the open folder to face the reporter and was indicating one page. "As far as I'm concerned, the case is closed. I was only doing this as a favor. I'm not getting paid anything for it. If you want to find her on your own, it's fine with me. I can give you what we have so far."

The reporter copied down the information about Gianna's biological mother. Maiden name: Tina Holder. Year of birth: 1959. An old address. A place of employment: Denny's Restaurant, Perris, California. Then they both stood up.

"I hope I'm wrong," Rutherford said. "I really do. I think

Gianna's a sweet girl, and I like Diana, too. I don't like to think she's exploiting the kid."

"Thanks for your time," the writer said, shaking again the big hand he offered. She remembered that she had brought a copy of the article written months before for the *Orange County Register*. She held it out hesitantly. "I wrote this about Gianna."

"Thanks, hon," he said. "I'll read it."

She had her doubts.

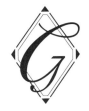

Confronting
the Doubts

All the way home from Pat Rutherford's office, the reporter's thoughts swirled. *Gianna not aborted after all? If Gianna wasn't aborted, there's no story!*

She couldn't help thinking what the radical leaders of the pro-choice movement would do with this. It would look like a deliberately perpetrated hoax—or at the least, like a cover-up. *They could smear the pro-life movement from here to the twenty-first century,* she thought, *and with some justification.* The best thing to do would be to announce that everyone had been genuinely mistaken but now wanted to correct the record.

Had Diana been genuinely mistaken? If she knew Gianna wasn't aborted, why had she told everyone she was? Why did she tell Gianna she was aborted and allow her to announce it at meetings?

Or had she lied? Was Diana sinister and devious? Even as these thoughts flooded the reporter's mind, the first flicker of anger gave way to amusement. *Diana, deceptive? No way.* Diana was one of the most open, engagingly honest people she'd ever met.

Besides, what did Diana have to gain by lying about Gianna's birth?

Attention. Publicity.

But negative publicity? Who would want to be labeled "a pro-life activist with a prop"?

Besides, *Diana* was the one who had initiated the search for Gianna's biological mother. Why would she insist on trying to find the very person who could prove her story false?

189

Okay, so maybe she didn't *know* it was false. The reporter tried to recall what Diana had said. Diana really believed the abortion story was true. Maybe someone had told her Gianna was aborted—her mother, maybe, or Gianna's caseworker. But why would anyone want her to think that if it weren't true?

Through the reporter's swirling thoughts came the dim memory of a document Diana had showed her. In fact, Diana had made her a copy of it and given it to her—tearing off the bottom of the sheet to protect the identity of the caseworker who had signed it. Wasn't it a medical record claiming Gianna was aborted?

As soon as she got home, the reporter dashed to her files. There it was, with MEDICAL INFORMATION printed at the top: "As natural mother gave date of 1/19/77 as last menstrual period, it was elected to do a saline abortion as natural mother wished to terminate the pregnancy." A typed physical description of the mother followed.

But there was no date on it and no name, either the name Giana or the name of the natural mother. It could have been the record of any one of the more than one million abortions done in 1977 after January 19—or at least one of the multitude of abortions done on white women 5'5½" tall, weighing 135 pounds, with brown hair and hazel eyes.

Was the reporter the victim of a false assumption?

Gianna's biological mother was the key to the truth—if she would *tell* the truth.

The reporter called the Denny's restaurant in Perris, a city east of Los Angeles, which had been written in Rutherford's files as the birth mother's workplace, and asked for Tina Holder. Tina no longer worked there. No, they didn't know where she had gone.

The reporter was not a private investigator. She had no idea where to take it from there. She gave up, put away her tape recorder and clipboard, and turned to other projects.

Then she received a letter from Rutherford. He had read

her article. "Now that I have read the story," he wrote, "I feel this girl is doing a great service to our God. . . . There's enough proof that what happened is true. . . . The Lord is telling me to stay on Gianna's side, and that is where my feet are planted. . . . I know the Lord has great things in store for Gianna."

It was the validation the reporter needed to continue her search. But how? Rutherford claimed he could find anyone in the world with only a name and a date of birth. She had more than that, but she wasn't sure how to follow it up.

Besides, she wasn't at all sure this woman wanted to be found. Would she herself, under similar circumstances? What if she did find Gianna's birth mother? What would keep her from hanging up the minute she heard the name Gianna? A door closed in their faces was a lot worse than a door that no one had yet knocked on.

Three weeks later, in March 1992, the reporter was still vacillating, wondering how and whether to invade this woman's life if she could be located, when Rutherford called.

"We've found Gianna's birth mom," he said excitedly, "and what a story! I talked to Tina this morning. She's married and living back here in Southern California. She called the abortion clinic a 'butcher shop.' She said Gianna came out squealing and hollering."

The reporter could almost see him shaking his head with amazement at the scene.

"She felt no remorse until she heard the baby cry. Something snapped in her when the baby cried. That got to her—she was brokenhearted!"

The reporter had no sooner hung up the phone with Rutherford than Rich Buhler, the radio talk-show host, called her. "I just talked to Tina," said Buhler. "What a sweet gal! She's lived life on the rough edge, but she loves the Lord, and she's fully pro-life. She feels she was a victim of the pro-abortionists. Said she would like to stand on the highest point of Washington, D.C., and tell them off!

"There's a lot she remembers—and a lot she doesn't. I don't know if it's because of the trauma or what. Filtering through all the hardships she's been through, she's really quite a bright person.

"She cries into her pillow over Gianna, prays for her, and loves her. She saw Gianna on 'The Maury Povich Show' and heard Gianna say that she wasn't sure she wanted to meet her mother. Tina doesn't want to enter Gianna's life till Gianna is ready for her to."

When Gianna learned her birth mother had been found and wanted to meet her, she said what she always had: "I don't feel a need to meet her. I forgive her, but I have my family. Ask her if she'll write to me instead."

When the reporter called Tina to see if she would be willing to talk about the abortion, she wasn't as open as she had been with Rutherford and Buhler. "I don't want to ever upset Gianna's life. I've already upset it enough. Before I tell any more of my story to anyone else, I want to tell her in person first."

The reporter relayed this to Gianna, who said candidly, "I can't sit down face to face with her. I just can't do it. I think it would be too much."

When the reporter called Tina to tell her this, she said, "My husband and I are moving again."

It seemed pushy to ask for the new address. "You have my number," the reporter said. "Call me when you get settled." But would she?

Whether she contacted them again or not, there was one thing about which all—Diana, Buhler, Rutherford, Tina, and the reporter—were agreed: As far as meeting with her birth mother was concerned, Gianna would call the shots. Nobody wanted her hurt.

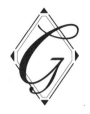

Tina's
Story

Tina didn't call when she got settled. After giving Rich Buhler and Pat Rutherford tantalizing bits of her story over the phone, she plunged into hiding, careful to keep out of the "system" Rutherford had used to trace her the first time.

It wasn't until April 1, 1993—more than a year later—that the reporter's home phone rang and a shaky voice on the other end said, "Hi. This is Tina."

Tina? The reporter's heart raced, but she forced herself to sound calm. "Hi, Tina. I've been hoping you'd call!"

"It's time. I need to face the past, and I've been putting it off for a year now. I feel like I can't breathe. It's so hard to know what to say."

The reporter's heart went out to her. "Take your time. I know it's taken a lot of courage to call."

"Breathe, Tina, breathe!" Tina told herself. The reporter could hear her let out her breath, trying to relax. "Dear God, help me!"

"Would you like to get together and talk?" the reporter asked. "I don't want to push you."

"I don't feel pushed. I feel guided."

A short time later, the reporter sat facing Tina across a booth in a Denny's restaurant. Tina's brown hair hung in soft waves past her shoulders, and she didn't look at all like the hard-bitten woman the reporter had expected. Like Gianna, she was, in fact, pretty.

"Do you want to talk about what happened?" the reporter asked.

Tina paused just a moment, and then she began. "It was a slaughterhouse," she said, having obviously given the experience a lot of thought. "It wasn't a hospital. Hospitals are where they take care of you. They bring life in a hospital. This was grotesque."

It was midafternoon, and they had the restaurant almost to themselves. The reporter sipped an iced tea and took notes as fast as she could, but Tina ignored her lemonade as the memories flooded back. "None of us there had any idea what abortion was. All we heard was that it was legal." She described the injection, the long wait, the birth. "I could have waited till everything froze over for that nurse.

"When Gianna was born"—Tina still pronounced the name with a hard G—"when her head came out and she was crying, I felt like it was meant to be. The first moment I felt her in my hands and saw her face and heard her cry, I knew what I did was so wrong. How could I ever do that? I was raised in two families, and in both I was loved—abortion was no part of that. I had my whole life mapped out, and it all fell apart in one day."

The story of her life spilled out as though she had to purge her conscience and this reporter offered the sympathetic ear she needed. First came the bare facts. Her father was an alcoholic. Her grandmother—"I called her Mom"—lived with the family in Anaheim, the same city where Diana had grown up. Tina was one of four kids, all of whom were dysfunctional.

She went on to describe two extremely painful childhood events. One was being molested by a family member. Then, on top of that, her parents divorced when she was ten.

Tina sought refuge from the hurt in her home by spending all the time she could with a friendly family across the street. "I'd think up excuses to visit them," she said, smiling at the memory. "I'd throw my shoes through their open window so I could knock on the front door and say, 'I left my shoes here last night.' I'd drop in and say hi before I went to school.

They loved me. There used to be presents for me under their Christmas tree."

But then this shelter in the storms of her young life threatened to disappear. "When I was eight, I dropped in on them, and Joyce, the mother, was packing. They were moving to Texas! She made the mistake of telling me, 'I wish I could put you in my pocket and take you along.' I ran home—my mom was on the phone—and I said, 'Get off the phone, I'm going to Texas!'

"My family let me go with them! Joyce's family treated me like their own child."

However, even a new, loving family and a move halfway across the country couldn't erase the lingering effects of the hurts she had already endured. "I thought, since I was molested as a child, that I deserved bad things. I was the best little Susie Homemaker—that's what they called me. I got off on cleaning and cooking. But I didn't feel it was enough. I felt I had to be perfect.

"Because of my feelings about the molestation, I gained a lot of weight. I moved into the pantry! I didn't talk; I ate and ate and ate. I went from an hourglass 70 pounds to 318 pounds. I found comfort in Twinkies."

Tina paused again, and her face grew clouded as she thought about what she was going to say next.

"When I was 15, Joyce got very sick and depressed. One day, I overheard her say, 'We should never have taken in a stray.' I'm sure she wouldn't have said it if she hadn't been feeling so bad, but I lost it. I walked out, and I haven't seen or talked to them since. I took to the streets and had a relationship with a guy who abused me. Then I went back to California."

Returning to her mother's home, Tina was in for a big and pleasant surprise.

"My mom had gained a lot of weight. I said, 'What are you, pregnant or something?' and she said, 'Yes!' When my little sister was born, I was so stoked. We became really close.

Amber is only two years older than Gianna, but she's Gianna's aunt. My eldest brother stopped doing drugs and got saved. We started going to church—we were all saved at that point."

Her new sister and new relationship with God gave Tina fresh motivation for living. Under a doctor's direction, she began to lose weight. "Every day I did 200 sit-ups, bends, and stretches. All I did all day was watch my little sister (who was about six months old) and exercise."

By the time she met Gianna's father, Tina had lost weight all the way down to 120 pounds. She was thrilled when the handsome young man took an interest in her. "He had green eyes and almost black hair. He was gorgeous. Today they'd call him a hunk."

She only knew him a couple of months, and he never learned she was pregnant. Her eyes misted over as she explained, "When I went to tell him, his apartment manager told me he had moved—and that he'd gotten another girl pregnant. He was an alcoholic, just like my father."

They had been talking three and a half hours. The reporter paid for the two beverages, left a large tip, and drove Tina to her apartment. When they got there, they sat in the car and resumed talking.

"How did you feel when you learned you were pregnant?" the reporter asked.

"I knew I was blessed with Gianna from the moment I conceived her. I had been using pot, but as soon as I got pregnant, I stopped immediately. I even became a vegetarian."

Unfortunately, some hard aspects of reality became clear not long after Tina got pregnant. She was living with her mother, younger brother, and baby sister. She had no job, and she couldn't get welfare because her mom did, and the state wouldn't send two welfare checks to the same address. She also didn't feel it was fair to the baby for her to be a welfare mother.

As the months went by, Tina had a growing conviction

that she just wasn't in a position to raise a child. She went to Planned Parenthood for help in deciding her best course of action. They reinforced all her fears about her ability to care for a baby and gave her no encouragement whatsoever to carry the baby to term. Eventually she concluded that her only choice was to abort. "Planned Parenthood had a lot to do with that," she said. "They were very convincing—they felt this was the best thing since tuna fish in a can."

After the abortion, however, Tina quickly grew attached to Gianna. The young mother couldn't wait for her new daughter to develop to the point of being ready to leave the hospital.

"Gianna went from the hospital to a foster home to me. She was almost five months old when I got her. I thought, *I'm bringing her home no matter what happens!* My mom took her to church all the time. She was their 'miracle baby.' I used to sing to her every day. We were very close, day and night— we did everything together."

Tina's mother, however, seemed convinced that they simply couldn't keep and care for Gianna. So she took drastic action, Tina believes, to have Gianna removed from the picture.

"One day I left my mom's home, and when I came back, Gianna was gone. My mother must have called Social Services. She had her own baby and had gone back to work, so she couldn't afford Gianna. I flipped out. Social Services told me I needed a two-bedroom apartment, a job, a 24-hour-a-day baby-sitter, and a car to take her to doctor's appointments—all that to support and keep her. They knew it was unrealistic and outrageous."

The loss of her daughter was the latest and greatest blow in Tina's still-young life. "I think it almost killed me when she was gone," she said, tears filling her eyes. "I was ecstatic with Gianna—when I was pregnant and when I was with her. She was the best thing that ever happened to me. And then she was gone."

Tina knew she couldn't meet the requirements imposed by Social Services for getting Gianna back. After a while, as she was still struggling with that harsh reality, the department asked her to sign some papers. Tina said she didn't know what they were, but they were, in fact, forms releasing Gianna for adoption.

"When I found out, I lost it again," Tina said, dabbing her eyes. "I thought I'd never see her again. I did see her once in her foster home in Cypress. It took everything out of me. I felt like a deflated balloon because she wasn't in my arms."

Tina desperately wanted to maintain contact with her daughter. While Gianna's presence had given her joy and love and hope just a short time before, now her absence left Tina in greater despair than ever. "I'd become accustomed to her smile. I used to look for her on playgrounds. I used to hear her cry—and she wasn't there," Tina said, gazing into the distance.

As much as she wanted to be with Gianna, however, the thought of going to see her in the foster home—and having to leave her there after a short visit—was almost too painful to bear. "After the first time, I *couldn't* go for more visits," she cried. "It was too hard on me!"

And so she disappeared from Gianna's life.

Gianna, however, had never left Tina's heart and mind. As the reporter sat with her in the car, it was clear that the pain of Tina's loss was still fresh after all those years.

"Every year on her birthday, I flip out again," Tina said, fighting to regain control of her emotions. "I cry a lot, buy her a card, and wish her happy birthday. Buying her cards and presents was my own secret no one ever knew about. I'd say the presents were for me, and they *were* for me, because she's a part of me."

Tina's hazel eyes filled with tears once more. "I couldn't relate. Why were there so many requirements for me to have her? *Other* people have kids and get welfare. Maybe it was because of the abortion. They probably thought, *She tried to kill her, so we can't leave her there.* I couldn't do anything about it."

The realization that Gianna was out of her life for good was emotionally devastating. Tina lost her will to live and soon began engaging in self-destructive behaviors.

"I did a lot of drugs," she said. "I tried to stay as high as I could for as many hours a day as I could. But no matter how much pot I smoked to numb my mind, I could never get her out of it. I already knew I did wrong for having the abortion. I was continually trying suicide through drugs. I deserved it. Sometimes I still feel that way."

During this period, however, Tina did meet, fall in love with, and marry another man. And her life started to turn around when she and her husband moved to Indiana to be near his dying mother. There she rediscovered God and the faith she had abandoned for a time.

"I got back with the Lord pretty strong in Indiana," Tina said simply. "I was growing before and after I saw her on 'The Maury Povich Show.' "

Suddenly she changed the subject as it dawned on her that she hadn't yet inquired about Gianna. "Is she happy?" she asked.

"Very happy."

Tina was silent a few minutes, and then she said, "It's like I've been in shock all these years. Don't get me wrong, I functioned. But it wasn't Tina that was doing things. She was just watching.

"My little sister, Amber, has been a replacement for Gianna—not in my heart, just in my life. But I still miss Gianna immensely—her face, her smile, her laugh. Her laugh was so infectious, it was scary. It was my own laugh I was hearing. She had the most beautiful blue eyes. . . . Somewhere within me, that pain is still there."

She stared out the window and sighed, caught up in the memory. "I've asked forgiveness, but it doesn't feel like enough. I *definitely* need forgiveness for the things I've thought about the abortionist. I would love to shut him down!

"Such memories, to be buried for so long . . ." She sighed again and seemed to come back to the present. "It's time to deal with the things I haven't dealt with. I want to start *living* and whatever comes with that.

"It feels good inside, though. I feel like I'm a sponge, and I've been absorbing all kinds of abuse and bad things. But tonight, finally talking about these things openly, it was all squeezed out! Now I can just absorb what I want to."

The conversation finally drew to a close, and Tina and the reporter went their separate ways. The next day, Tina called the reporter to say, "Isn't it a *beautiful* day? I feel so free! It's like I'm a child again—and it's okay! For the first time, my happiness is greater than my guilt!"

Tina and Diana met over breakfast in the same booth at the same Denny's restaurant a few days later. They were as friendly and casual as if they'd grown up together. "The memories!" said Tina, marveling. "It's like a floodgate is opened and I'm not in control of the levers anymore. So much is coming back!" She asked Diana, "Is there anything you want to know?"

Diana asked about where Tina grew up in Anaheim, and they reminisced about pre-Disneyland days. Then Tina told about her dysfunctional past and her abusive relationships. "It's like for years, I've just accepted all the you-know-what to take care of the guilt."

"You felt you deserved it."

"Oh, yes. And now I'm out of jail."

"I know what you mean," said Diana. "I've had to deal with my own share of guilt."

"But I'm not concerned about the future. I'm just enjoying the moment."

"Well, what shall I tell you about Gianna?"

"I don't know where to begin. I have a million questions. I feel the Lord blessed me with you. You are heaven-sent. I made a deal with God that if I let her go, He would put Gianna in a place where she would be totally loved—unconditionally."

"She has that," said Diana.

"It's apparent. It oozes out of you."

"She's a special kid."

"From the moment I conceived, I knew I was pregnant. I wanted her. I felt so glorious inside. I knew she was a miracle."

"I brought Gianna up with the idea that you were deceived," said Diana.

"I *was* deceived by Planned Parenthood. The whole thing was the most bizarre line: 'You don't need this. You don't want this. Let us *help* you!' Incredibly crafted lines. I would love to shut them all down.

"Gianna was kicking and acting normal right through the saline. It didn't faze her. She was just loving life. My body and her body totally rejected the chemicals. We had bonded. We had super rapport by then—there was no way she was going to die! We were both too strong-willed.

"Her birth was a joyous occasion for me. I was so cool and calm, like that was the way it was supposed to happen. But for the other girls there, they wanted it to be *their* baby."

"They were faced with reality," said Diana.

"Yeah, slam-bam!" Tina paused for a moment, then added, "I've prayed for them."

They both sat, musing.

"Gianna looked like a little, wet rag—with hair!" marveled Tina. "I saw her later in the hospital, and then she came to live with me and my mother and brother and sister. I was so stoked I couldn't see straight. I knew I'd been blessed immensely. She came to the land of chaos, but she was the brightest light shining."

Tina then retold the story of how she lost custody of Gianna and how that made her feel. "I don't think I've ever really dealt with that," she said. "They should have taken care of me—of *this* child—and then Gianna would have been all right."

Diana looked at her sympathetically. "*You* were the one who needed foster care. If they had rescued *you*, they would have rescued both of you."

They had been talking for nearly four hours. After they paid the bill and walked outside, Gianna's two mothers hugged each other. And then, much as she had after unburdening herself to the reporter, Tina exclaimed, "Isn't it the most gorgeous day?"

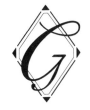

Becoming a Young Woman

Almost two years after going to Amy Grant's home outside Nashville, only to find she was out of town, Gianna returned from a tour to tell her friends elatedly, "I finally met Amy Grant!" They were both at a fundraiser in Tennessee. When they were introduced, Amy said to Gianna, "You're the one who came to my house and wrote me a really nice note!" It was the first time Gianna had felt absolutely speechless. "I felt so shy, I turned around and ran away!" Talking about it, she put her hands to her mouth in embarrassment.

After the program, Gianna had gone up on stage and told Amy she would pray for her, and Amy had responded with a hug.

The two were scheduled to share the stage at the Creation Festival in Mount Union, Pennsylvania. "There will be 50,000 people there," Gianna announced. But that didn't seem to awe her as much as the fact that "I'll be on stage right before Amy Grant! I get to be backstage with her!"

Early in 1993, Diana became friends with the mother of a girl Gianna's age. The girl's name was Rachel Oliver (no relation to Jessi Oliver). Rachel remembers her first meeting with Gianna:

"I saw the article about Gianna in *Brio* a month before, and I was real intimidated, so I didn't talk to her. I got along better with her sister and her mom." Before long, however, the girls hit it off. They found they both liked eating at the same Italian restaurant. "Gianna likes to embarrass me by always asking for Tabasco sauce and jalapeño peppers. She puts them on everything," Rachel says. "She got me hooked on hazelnut coffee and iced mochas."

On June 26, 1993, Gianna, Jenny Morson, and Rachel attended the Creation Festival in Pennsylvania to which Gianna had been looking forward.

"It was like a combination Christian Woodstock and a carnival," Rachel said afterward. "People brought their kids and camped in a big field for a week."

Gianna couldn't get over her excitement at getting to hear and meet all her favorite singers: DC Talk, Out of the Grey, Prayer Chain. She wasn't scheduled to sing, but she was going to have an opportunity to say a few words—not to the 50,000 she had expected, which was intimidating enough, but to 65,000 people. Public speaking had become second nature to her, but 65,000 people! For once, Gianna wrote out what she wanted to say ahead of time and memorized it.

She didn't tell the story of her birth this time. She talked about being happy to be at the same conference as Amy Grant, about abstinence, about making a stand, and about how each person can make a difference. Amy Grant sang later that evening. It was an event Gianna will always remember.

Rachel was able to take trips with Gianna in 1993 to Pennsylvania (including a tour through the Hershey chocolate factory) and New Hampshire. In October, Gianna performed at a church in Michigan, and afterward she and Diana got to drive slowly along the shore of Lake Michigan and revel in the autumn colors.

In January 1994, Gianna and Diana appeared with pro-life physician Dr. John Willke and Concerned Women for America president Beverly LaHaye in a video, *Winning the War on the Unborn*, produced by the Institute for Creation Research in El Cajon, California.

"I picture the Lord's strong hand always covering me and not letting me be harmed," Gianna said of her biological mother's abortion. "Her sin nearly killed me, but my sin did kill Jesus, and I've been forgiven on the cross, so I can forgive her also.

"I talk to women every day who say, 'Why didn't someone tell me? I have nightmares about the situation.' Post-abortion trauma is remembering and grieving for your child. Really the only way you can be set free from this is through the cross of Christ. You can put these things at the foot of the cross and ask Him to heal you and help you move on."

Men need forgiveness, too, Gianna said, if they helped a girlfriend get an abortion. "Every person who is around this is somehow affected by it."

Diana agreed. "I'm concerned for teens that have had siblings aborted before or after them. Surviving twins have a tremendously hard time dealing with that. And grandparents have a major loss when grandchildren are aborted."

In keeping with the institute's commitment to creation science, interviewer Pat Loy's questions sought a link between abortion and evolution.

"I have some miscarried babies, from the first trimester to 22 weeks, preserved in formaldehyde," Diana said. "I took them with me when I gave pro-life talks. Schoolchildren never related to them as a fish. They could tell they were babies."

"I was speaking in this crowd of people at this college campus," put in Gianna. "I was getting these *really* tough questions, and it didn't dawn on me that a lot of the crowd was pro-abortion and they were just giving me all these twisted, complicated questions. There was no way I could answer them without the help of God. I mean, the answers were just coming, and it was like, 'Whoa, where did I get that?' you know. It was really God.

"This one woman was talking about how babies in the womb are like fish, and I just went, 'I am not a fish; I was not a fish; I was a human being. I didn't come out as a swimming, wobbling fish but as a human being baby—crying and screaming very loudly.' "

She gave listeners another, sobering perspective on the issue: "People don't realize that the abortion industry is a money-making industry. The bigger the baby, the more money people may make. You don't hear that when you hear about women's choice."

Gianna had met Josh McDowell in the summer of 1993. They were both sitting in a trailer, waiting to go onstage at the Fishnet Festival in Virginia, where Gianna was going to sing "Amazing Grace." McDowell, author of 40 books including *Why Wait?* has had an effective ministry promoting chastity among high-school and college students.

McDowell and Gianna were instant friends, and he had no trouble persuading her to grant him an interview with cohost Wayne Shepherd for Josh McDowell Radio. The interview aired on March 12, 1994, when Gianna was 16.

Gianna's enthusiasm was evident from her squeal, almost overloading the mikes, in answer to the first question. "I guess you can tell I'm excited," she said with a laugh. Her exuberance and lack of guile seemed to touch the hearts of the two men interviewing her.

There were the usual questions about the abortion and her cerebral palsy. "You're very active. I understand you play softball."

"I used to," Gianna corrected them. "This is my activity now: sitting on an airplane and running through airports."

McDowell and Shepherd asked Gianna about her ministry to teens.

"To the kids I'm trying to reach every day," Gianna said, "[abortion] is a woman's right, [the baby] is just a blob. So what I do is just say, 'Look, I was not a blob. I was the baby that you're saying it's a woman's right to kill.'

"It's frustrating because it's hard to get through to them sometimes, but I just pray for the words and love them as much as I can."

"You travel and sing and speak," McDowell said. "What

do you tell people when you speak to groups?"

"Well, first of all, I'm bringing the gospel message. I think there are so many pro-lifers that can get so caught up in the emotion of the abortion issue that sometimes they forget that the number one message that we're to bring is the gospel. So I bring that first, and the abortion issue I bring in (through) my testimony. But really I have a heart for teenagers. I talk a lot about abstinence and the purity ring that James Dobson promotes—I have one myself. My main message, though, is a message of forgiveness."

They asked Gianna about Operation Rescue. "What feelings go through you, as an abortion survivor, when you see men and women out there taking a stand, being arrested?"

"I've been arrested myself," Gianna said candidly. "I know that's a very controversial issue, but I'm just being honest with you. I have been to rescues before—many—and when I see it on the news, it's not at all portrayed truthfully. What's portrayed is the radical pro-lifers that don't have a clue about what's going on and [are] just traumatizing women. What I've seen when I go to a rescue is Christians lovingly sitting at a door and talking to the women about to go in, saying, 'This is what you're doing. Let me help you. Let me take you to a crisis pregnancy center.' They do get arrested for it, that's true, of course, because right now it's against the law.

"I'm not involved with Operation Rescue, but I am involved with a group called Youth for America Missionaries to the Pre-born, and they just really have hearts for God, and they're true missionaries, I believe. If you could see *that* on the news, I think it would really change people's view."

They asked, "Why do you think God saved you and not other babies?"

Gianna hesitated. "That's a difficult question to answer, because I'm not God. I really don't know why God chose to spare my life and not others, but I do believe that I have a purpose on this earth, and that is to tell people about Jesus in the most loving way I can. And I do believe that the children who are aborted go directly into the arms of Jesus."

"What's God teaching you right now?"

"That if you're a soldier and you get wounded, you can't lay down and die, but you have to stand back up and fight."

"What's your favorite scripture?"

"Jeremiah 1. He's very encouraging to me, because Jeremiah was young when God called him, and he said, 'Lord, I can't do this,' and the Lord said, 'Yes, you can. I'm going to be with you.' And Philippians 2, all about Christ's humility, that He is God but He is so humble."

On a lighter note, they asked if Gianna had a boyfriend, and she said with feeling, "Oh, I want one so bad! I do!"

"Typical 16-year-old!" the men responded, laughing. "Maybe we have someone listening right now who would like to apply!" McDowell told her, "You'll make quite a catch."

McDowell closed the broadcast with a prayer thanking God "for bringing such a wonderful, spirited sister into our lives" and asking Him "to bring her to maturity and use her to reach other teenagers."

As he finished, still on the air, Gianna told McDowell, "I really appreciate all that you do, too. You're just an awesome guy. What can I say?"

That same month, Gianna appeared on TBN. She spoke about Proverbs 6:16, which lists "six things the Lord hates, seven that are detestable to him." One of them is "hands that shed innocent blood." But she didn't focus on the negative. "My mom told me, 'Instead of concentrating on the fact that you almost died, praise God for the fact that you are alive.'

"I went through a long, hard time of 'Why did my birth mother give me up? What was wrong with me?' Mom always said, 'He loves you just the way you are.' Just knowing I was so loved by Jesus is what got me through—and knowing that the Lord could still use me, despite a disability, and that God placed me in the family He wanted me to be in. Now I don't have a desire to be healed of this disability."

Millions of Americans have seen Gianna, blonde hair rippling to her shoulders, singing in a choir in a 30-second TV spot—this despite the fact that every major American network refused to sell air time for its nonconfrontational message. Produced by the Arthur S. DeMoss Foundation as one of a series of tasteful ads showing children being valued by adults, the spot ends with the words: "Life. What a beautiful choice."

On April 20, 1994, Nancy DeMoss, chairman of the board of the foundation, and Cardinal John O'Connor received awards at the National Right to Life's First Annual Proudly Pro-Life Banquet for their efforts on behalf of unborn life. On receiving his award, the cardinal spoke of abortion as one of the twentieth century's examples of mass annihilation. In earlier holocausts, he pointed out, victims were those with the "wrong" religion or ethnic background. But with abortion, he said, "life itself has become the enemy." He added, "What in God's name could anyone with any sense of decency be but pro-life?"

Also at that dinner, Congressman Henry Hyde pointed out that pro-lifers are the only "special interest group" whose "special interest" is not *self*-interest. Gianna sang "Amazing Grace" for the 1,100 attending the banquet, among them Eunice Kennedy Shriver, actress Patricia Neal, governors and ambassadors, as well as 230 future leaders from the Northeast's finest colleges.

Despite the notables present, despite the fact that the event filled the Grand Ballroom of the Waldorf-Astoria Hotel in New York City, and despite the fact that C-SPAN covered a breakfast a few days later where an abortion rights group honored a senator for his support, not one major network mentioned the Proudly Pro-Life Banquet.

On May 22, when Gianna and Diana returned from a concert in Durham, North Carolina, Dené met them with the sad news that Grandpa John had passed away the day

before at the age of 104. He had been living in a convalescent home since suffering a stroke.

"I've been expecting it," Diana said sadly. "The last time I
visited him, I fed him yogurt, and he kept falling asleep." That
visit had been two weeks earlier, the day before the trip east.

"I'm *so* glad Jessi and I changed our minds and came in to
see him that last time," Gianna said with feeling. She told
Dené, "We were sitting in the car while Mom was seeing
Grandpa, and suddenly we just decided to go in and see him,
too. I would have felt terrible if I hadn't seen him one more
time."

Diana lacked the money for a nice coffin, so she reluc-
tantly had Grandpa's body cremated instead. One of the
handful of people who attended his funeral was a fellow street
person who remembered that Grandpa had once given him a
bag of sweet potatoes. They buried Grandpa's ashes under a
tree in a cemetery in Escondido.

When summer came, Gianna tried something new. She
had talked to Rachel about wanting to dye her hair.

"Would *you* do it?" Gianna asked.

"Never!" Rachel declared.

"I would."

When Gianna called to tell her she had a surprise for her,
Rachel guessed at once.

"What color?"

"Black cherry. Well, it was *supposed* to be black cherry. It's
more like—well, just come over and see."

"It's more like purple," Diana told Rachel, meeting her at
the door. Gianna had talked Dené into doing it for her, and
they had used permanent dye.

Despite all attempts to recover her natural color, Gianna
spent the summer of 1994 with purple hair. At her first prom
and as bridesmaid in Dené's wedding on June 11, wearing her
first high heels, her hair was still causing double takes.

Gianna had said in her interview with Josh McDowell, "I
love to hang out with friends and be with my sister. My sister

and I have been extremely close. She's 21. We didn't used to be so close, but now we are, and she's just one of my best friends."

Diana credited Dené with discipling Gianna: "She had a lot to do with making Gianna what she is today. They're good buddies."

Neither Gianna's schedule nor Dené's wedding interfered with that. She and Gianna still keep in touch through frequent phone calls, letters, and funny cards. Dené's schooling (after earning an AA degree in theology, she is getting a degree in graphic arts) prevented her from accompanying Gianna on her concert tours, although they did spend a two-week vacation in Austria together. But Dené says she doesn't feel left out. "I've never felt deprived or cheated. I'm a behind-the-scenes person anyway. That's how I want it. Gianna's always been really, really special, my best friend."

At her concerts for the rest of the summer, where Gianna had to keep explaining her hair, she was more popular than ever. Teens crowded around her to say, "We love your hair! How can we do ours like that?"

Meanwhile, their mothers would seek out Diana to ask anxiously, "Doesn't that bother you?"

Diana would reassure them, "It's not her heart. It's just her hair."

Eventually, when they came home, Gianna would spend 11 hours in a beauty shop, having her hair bleached and having blonde woven back into it.

For part of the summer, Gianna's left leg was in a cast again. With new growth, the spastic muscles in her leg were making her walk on tiptoe once more. But that didn't slow her down. She sang and gave her testimony at Church on the Way, pastored by Jack Hayford, in Van Nuys, California, the week after Dené's wedding. She helped record an abstinence video for teens, *3D—A Pledge to Purity*, with Lisa Whelchel from "Facts of Life," right after spending a week at her first youth retreat.

Gianna's favorite thing to do when she's home is to go to youth group. As she told one interviewer, "That's what I live and die for. I *gotta* go!"

"Youth group" was the high-school and young college group Rachel attended at Pacific Hills Church in Aliso Viejo. When she was on the road, Gianna would sometimes call Tim Hahne, the youth pastor, to discuss what she was going through and ask for advice or prayer.

In August, Tim and five other adults and 43 kids were going to Sequoia National Park. Gianna especially wanted to go on the retreat, because she had never been on one before—she had always been out of town.

"Gianna was a real trooper," says Tim. "We hiked a lot, and there wasn't anyplace she didn't go with us." They hiked along the Kaweah River and slid down natural rock slides, landing in waterfalls. They saw black bears. While hiking on a steep hill behind their campsite with a girlfriend and two guys, Gianna slipped and fell into a hornet's nest. She and the two boys, who came to her rescue, each got stung several times.

Gianna remembers that incident fondly. "It was *great*," she says. "I mean, at least I tried hiking, and I was with people I love."

There were Bible studies in the mornings. In the evenings, Tim and two other pastors gave a series of talks on becoming "a vessel of honor fit for the Master's use" from the book of 2 Timothy. Teams of students, eight guys and eight girls, would take turns preparing meals for the whole group and would pray with each other at bedtime.

Pastor Tim planned to baptize some of the students in the river, and he extended the invitation to anyone who wanted to be baptized again. "It isn't necessary," he told them, "but if you were baptized when you were very young, you may want to do it again, now that you understand its significance."

Gianna was one of 13 who decided to be baptized again. On a hot day, everyone piled into cars and drove a half hour down the mountain to the Buckeye swimming hole on the Kaweah River where they had played on the rock slides. Surrounded by forest, the pool was calm, although the sounds of the river babbling farther on filled the air with melody.

In bathing suit and shorts, Gianna waded out to Tim when her turn came. She explained to him why she wanted to be baptized, and Tim repeated her words in a shout so they could be heard over the noise of the river.

"I want to be baptized again because I was really young the first time," Gianna said. "I didn't know what it meant. Now I know that it's a way to tell the world that I've confessed I'm a sinner and turned away from my sins, and I've trusted in Jesus to be my Savior and the Lord of my life. I'm publicly identifying with His death for my sins, His burial, and His resurrection. I love Him with all my heart! The setting here is so beautiful, too, and being with my friends is so special."

Tim dunked her under the water, and when she came up, radiant, everyone clapped.

What Gianna liked most about the retreat, she told Pastor Tim afterward, was the fact that people treated her normally. Not as an abortion survivor. Not as a disabled person. Just as a sister in the Lord.

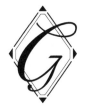

What's Next?

chapter 23

Life has come full circle. Gianna is 17 at the time of this writing, the age her birth mother was when she took the long, lonely bus ride into Los Angeles to abort her. Gianna mentions this occasionally in her talks, saying, "I think of it sometimes and wonder what it must have been like for her."

She handles debates with equanimity now, no longer afraid of pro-abortionists. Her fear peaked when she started to meet some of them and feel the brunt of their hostility. For months, she dreamed that angry women were chasing her, shouting, "There's a survivor! Get her! Get her!"

Diana spent a lot of time with Gianna, talking about the nightmares and praying with her for God to take the fear away. "If they were going to 'get' anyone," Diana said, "it would be me, not you."

One day Gianna told her mother, "God did it! The dreams are gone! I'm not afraid anymore!" Neither the fears nor the nightmares have returned.

During a recent phone interview, broadcast live, a radio host patched through to Gianna's home a call from a man who saw nothing wrong with abortion.

"I wasn't a baby?" Diana heard Gianna ask incredulously. "Then what was I—a fish?" Gianna seemed to be listening for a moment, and then she burst out, "A *collection* of *tissue?* That's a joke and a half! If I was part of my biological mother's body, I would have come out an organ."

There was silence again, and then she asked, more quietly, "So would you rather I hadn't survived? Oh, you're

221

glad I did?"

When she hung up, she was smiling. "These things don't bother me like they used to," she told her mom. "I kind of enjoy them."

Gianna and her mother still travel constantly on behalf of the gospel of Jesus Christ, the unborn, sexual abstinence, and pro-life and pro-family issues. Gianna continues writing and singing her own songs as well. Nine of them—blues, country, acoustic, and pop—are on her first album, "For the Sake of Love," which has sold well since its release in November 1993. She's getting ready to produce another.

At the time of this writing, after attending airplane school ("Delta Academy, United Academy, American Academy," as she puts it) for so many years, Gianna is preparing for the high-school equivalency exam, as well as her driver's test. She and Diana divide their time between ministry travel, San Clemente, and Franklin, Tennessee (near Nashville), where they live on two and a half acres in the country. Their ministry, Alive! Ministries, is also headquartered in Franklin. Gianna is making friends in her new community.

"Once no one wanted to hang out with me," she says. "Now I have friends all around the world."

She wants to attend Belmont University in Nashville in the near future, majoring—of course—in music. Jessi would like to enroll, too, and they could room together.

Gianna also wants to work with The Bridge, a youth outreach of Calvary Chapel in Franklin, Tennessee. She wants to do "more stuff for teens" in the area of chastity and abstinence.

Diana has always dreamed of opening a home for unwed mothers. She supports Joshua's House, a shelter for unwed mothers in Covina, California, run by Compassion Network. With Gianna in college soon and Dené married, she hopes to start a foundation that would make possible nationwide shelters. She also oversees the women's ministries of Calvary Chapel in Franklin. "My heart has always been in service," she says.

Penny is still taking in high-risk and hard-to-place children, most of them under the age of three. Many of them are cocaine-addicted newborns. Sooner or later, they all find a permanent home.

Penny's low, mint-green house in Anaheim has a big backyard covering half an acre, surrounded by a chain-link fence. For years, she has dreamed of adding on to it to form six bedrooms, all opening into an enormous playroom. There would be two foster children to a room, with supervisors to care for them.

On other days she says, "I'm going to quit! I'm over 70. I'm too old for this!"

The caseworkers at Orange County Social Services tease her: "You said you were quitting two years ago!"

"Well, I might take a year off." But then, if she took a year off, she just might use the time to build the playroom.

The doctor who aborted Gianna now owns 46 clinics throughout the Southwest. He is still doing abortions.

To contact Gianna Jessen for information about her concerts and other ministry opportunities, write to or call the following:

Alive! Ministries
P.O. Box 987
Franklin, TN 37065
(615) 794-2964

Afterword

We would like to thank Dr. James Dobson and Focus on the Family for their efforts with this book and for their uncompromising stand for life. We also extend our love to the people of America and beyond who, through prayer and grassroots efforts, make known the value of life and the glory of its Giver.

We are forever grateful to our pastors, Danny Bond of Pacific Hills Church in Aliso Viejo, California, and Alan Curtis of Calvary Chapel in Franklin, Tennessee. They instruct us soundly in the Word of God, pray for us as we step out in ministry, and never lose faith in the gospel of Jesus Christ. We're also thankful for those church fellowships, particularly the women's and youth ministries, which have surrounded us with prayer.

Next, we want to express our appreciation to the directors, staff, volunteers, and financial supporters of crisis pregnancy centers and shelter/shepherding homes everywhere. Those wonderful places serve both mothers and fathers in crisis pregnancies, as well as their children and families. The efforts of the people who make those centers possible encourage us to keep on keeping on. May God bless them abundantly in their labor for Him.

Finally, for our family and friends who have stood with us in the battle, we pray that God's love will always surround you and that His unspeakable joy will be written visibly on your lives.

Gianna Jessen and Diana De Paul
2 Corinthians 4

Focus on the Family Publications

Focus on the Family

This complimentary magazine provides inspiring stories, thought-provoking articles, and helpful information for families interested in traditional, biblical values. Each issue also includes a "Focus on the Family" radio broadcast schedule.

Parental Guidance

Close-ups and commentaries on the latest music, movies, television, and advertisements directed toward young people. Parents, as well as youth leaders, teachers, and pastors, will benefit from this indispensable newsletter.

All magazines are published monthly except where otherwise noted. For more information regarding these and other resources, please call Focus on the Family at (719)531-5181, or write to us at Focus on the Family, Colorado Springs, CO 80995.

Leanne
Kaye
Boyd
Please
Rear
To
Leanne
Kaye
Boyd

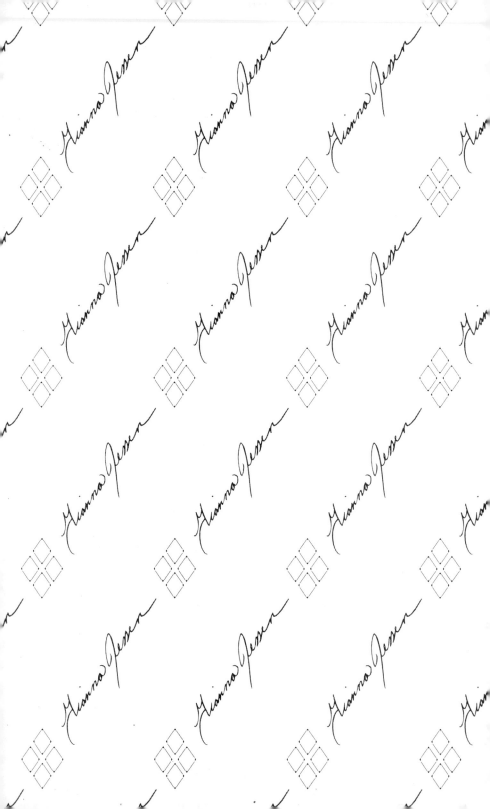